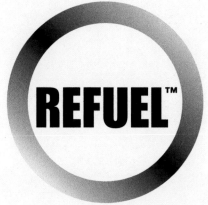

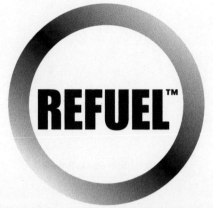

REFUEL™

A 24-Day Eating Plan to Shed Fat, Boost Testosterone, and Pump Up Strength and Stamina

JOHN LA PUMA, M.D.

with Gretchen Lees

HARMONY
BOOKS · NEW YORK

Published in the United States by Harmony Books, an imprint of the Crown Publishing Group,
a division of Random House LLC, a Penguin Random House Company, New York.
www.crownpublishing.com

Harmony Books is a registered trademark and the
Circle colophon is a trademark of Random House LLC.

Library of Congress Cataloging-in-Publication Data

La Puma, John.
Refuel : a 24-day eating plan to shed fat, boost testosterone,
and pump up strength and stamina / John La Puma, M.D.—First edition.
    pages   cm
Includes bibliographical references.
I. Reducing diets—Recipes.   2. Men—Health and hygiene—Popular works.
3. Testosterone—Popular works.   I. Title.
RM222.2.L34I4 2013
613.2'5—dc23
2012049788

ISBN 978-0-7704-3746-6
eBook ISBN 978-0-7704-3747-3

Printed in the United States of America

Book design: Ruth Lee-Mui
Jacket design: Michael Nagin
Jacket photography: Mickey Cashew / Getty Images

I 3 5 7 9 I0 8 6 4 2

First Edition

To David, whose life choices and words showcase the best of the modern healthy man. And to those who've signed up for my newsletter and discovered more book bonuses, tips, and tools on www.drjohnlapuma.com: May you become healthier, happier, and even more awesome, and help others do the same.

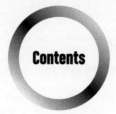

Contents

PART FOUR: GET REAL
The Simple Path to Enjoying the Food You Love

PART FIVE: FINAL THOUGHTS
Men Don't Diet. Men Refuel.

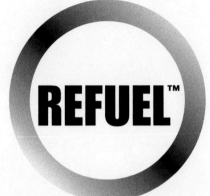

A DOCTOR'S MISSION FOR MEN

Brad is 59 years old and a successful software engineer. He is smart, quiet, accomplished, and very well respected. He has a great medical team ready to help with any health-related issue. He is 5 foot 7 inches and weighs 222 pounds.

Ten years ago he had prostate cancer, which was treated with hormonal therapy and radiation. Since then, he'd gained 20 pounds on top of the 30 pounds he'd previously accumulated as he embraced the lifestyle of a typical senior executive. With an extremely demanding work schedule and late nights, he was left with little time or energy to think about his own health and needs.

Recently his cardiologist had added a third cholesterol medicine. His trim, superfit wife worried that she would lose him, had begun to ask if he really needed that second glass of wine or the dessert at their favorite restaurant. He didn't, but it was habit, and he liked it.

He came to see me because his doctor told him he should, and because he had two goals. "I'd like to be in the top quartile for health for my age," he said. "And I'd like to avoid having to sing at the Christmas party." He'd made a bet with his best friend at work that he could lose 25 pounds by April 25. It was January 11.

Brad normally worked out with his trainer three mornings per week, and he ate cold cereal, eggs, juice, and toast for breakfast. At lunch, he had whatever was in the break room—usually pizza, and sometimes a salad. He worked late, except when there was an event, or he and his wife ate out (weekends and often during the week). When he was home, his wife made his favorites—steak, potatoes, chicken—and served meals on some of their large, beautiful plates. He favored desserts soaked in Grand Marnier. He rarely cooked, except occasionally to grill. He awoke early, ahead of the alarm, and went to sleep late. He didn't smoke, and never had. He drank a bottle of good wine at home weekly, and above all else, he treasured the flavor of hearty food and the feel of hard work.

"Don't give me food I can't eat," he said to me. "It's got to taste great or I won't eat it." Brad squirmed in his chair as he talked. He was in pain, because his belly overhung his belt and his back was in spasm. He couldn't do a pushup, a burpee, a squat, or a lunge. He was a little short of breath.

Brad was like too many of my patients: overworked, chronically stressed, and not producing at optimal levels, and with the abnormal laboratory tests, back pain, and elastic-waist sweatpants to show for it. Too often, men like Brad have an outsized tolerance for ignoring high blood pressure, high blood sugar, and high cholesterol. That hellish trinity creates impotence and heart failure, metabolic syndrome and stroke, but no man thinks about that while he's inhaling a hamburger, or trying not to spill the cup-holder of fries in his lap while driving home from work.

Most men, like Brad, are not following an exercise or diet program that works. If they're lucky enough to have a doctor who says, "Lose some weight," they make an initial effort to diet, but they usually fall off the wagon before long. They end up holding a carton of ice cream in their lap at night, instead of their partner. No amount of goading from their doctor or their partner or helpful family member helps.

But there's a way out for the Brads of the world. It's as practical and as methodical as it sounds, and it works: take one step, and then another. The success of the plan is incremental, and even a little success will spike your confidence and motivation to take the next step. Plan on succeeding—because other men have.

Brad began to do just that. He set small goals, every day, and did his best to achieve them. He didn't give up. And neither should you.

I didn't prescribe a diet for Brad, because diets have not worked for men (or for most women, for that matter). But I did give him the plan that I designed *specifically* for men. It is based on three strategic factors for men: their unique metabolism, mindset, and objectives.

Brad implemented a direct and tactical approach to achieving his health goals. His results: he became fit, lost weight, dropped several of his medications, and recovered his strength and stamina . . . to the tune of routinely running 7.5-minute miles and pumping out 12 pull-ups afterward.

Brad is one of many men I've treated over the last fifteen years who have come to me for help with weight and health management. Most of these guys walk into my Chef Clinic® feeling frustrated and somewhat defeated, but they walk out with a sustainable, practical approach to their health, and a tangible strategy that gives them a re-newed sense of confidence. Many of them feel as though a doctor is speaking with them directly for the first time—that they're getting a program tailor-made for their needs. They are. And the good news is that their experience can now be yours.

In *Refuel*™, I am making my plan available to the public for the first time. At www.drjohnlapuma.com, there are tools to test your testosterone, extra resources to boost it, and new ways to improve your skills and fitness naturally, plus man-to-man advice on food, fit-ness, cooking, and the plan itself. I've approached *Refuel* with my doctor's brain and my chef's taste buds; I've studied the best available research with an eye for cutting-edge information; and I've tested the plan on men who were interested in but not sold on it. Remarkably, they've experienced success—dropping their belly fat; lowering their blood pressure, cholesterol, and blood glucose levels; rediscovering real erections; reviving sex drive; getting leaner and stronger; and like Brad, regaining control of their lives. Now *Refuel* is available to you. It's time for you to take back control.

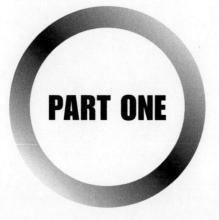

PART ONE

THE HEALTH CRISIS

The Unique Challenges You Face

1

THE BIOLOGY OF WEIGHT AND SEX

Why a Generic Weight-Loss Approach Does Not Work for You

When I first met Brad, I realized his health concerns might have become mine if I had not changed the course of my life years earlier, when I was in my early thirties and was accelerating along the fast track of my medical career. I was flying high professionally, but I wasn't taking care of myself. I inhaled highly processed foods mindlessly at work: bags of bagels and pints of cream cheese, egg rolls, doughnuts, pizza. I grabbed whatever I could eat and kept moving.

I tried to weekend-warrior my way out of my weight, but that of course didn't work. So there I was: 35 pounds overweight, with many of the early symptoms of aging. I noticed newly sprouting gray hair, I had a big gut, and I didn't like what I saw in the mirror. My uncle had died of diabetes at age 48, and I was starting to pee more and felt hungry all the time. I knew that I could be developing diabetes and that what I was eating was aging me, physically and mentally. But I didn't know how to stop the process, let alone reverse it.

On top of wanting to change for myself, I also felt a responsibility to change for my patients. How could I help them effectively when I couldn't make improvements in my own life?

THE FAT DOCTOR PARADOX

Ever been startled by the sight of a doctor lighting up? I have. But does the sight of an obese doctor give you the same jolt? It should.

Researchers with Johns Hopkins University's Bloomberg School of Public Health revealed in a study that a physician's weight can impact the type of care and information he or she issues to patients. After surveying doctors across the country, they found "normal-weight physicians" were more likely to discuss weight loss, diet, and exercise with their heavy patients. Only 7 percent of overweight physicians (individuals with a body mass index, or BMI, of 25 or more) recorded an obesity diagnosis on any patient versus 93 percent of normal-weight doctors.

My own research in this area reveals that doctors face huge challenges in the workplace. Free meals are in constant supply at many hospitals. Nutritional quality is not always considered—and I am being generous in my assessment here. To be more accurate, most hospital food seems designed to cause heart disease and other illness, not to prevent it.

By no means does this cancel out the care you receive from an overweight doctor or a fast-food-franchise-hosting hospital. But it does bring to light the fact that doctors are far from perfect, and that acquiring or building upon your self-care survival skills is never a bad idea.

I knew enough about the science of aging and weight gain to recognize that nutrition (or lack of it) had landed me in my current state, so I went straight to the source: food. But I didn't want to simply put on my medical scientist's hat. I wanted to learn a new skill: to understand food from a tactile sense, to use natural ingredients in their natural form. I wanted to approach food as a chef would, so I did the most obvious thing: I went to cooking school.

In cooking, I found a creative professional niche that also helped serve my personal goals. I was eating better than ever—in both taste and nutrition—and my body, appearance, and energy level reflected this change. I lost most of my big gut, and many of the external signs of aging that had begun to reveal themselves prematurely retreated. I felt my sense of purpose renewed.

> **HOT TIP**
> Soft, smooth skin and diminished underarm hair can signal low testosterone.

From there, and with my friend Dr. Mike Roizen, I became the first physician to teach nutrition and cooking together in a medical school. We went on to research and co-write a popular book, *The RealAge Diet*.

I took this momentum to re-invent my individual practice, Chef Clinic®, where I began to offer patients my hands-on, strategic plan for achieving better health through weight loss. I started collecting good stories, and writing down the details of my calls from patients. They were losing weight and doing things that they had never thought about doing. A few examples:

- A 72-year-old from Washington, D.C., called me after reaching the bottom of the Grand Canyon, over nine miles from where he had begun.
- A 54-year-old let me know he no longer needed to use seat belt extenders, and had to push his car's driver's seat forward because it was too far from the steering wheel.
- A 48-year-old had to take two links out of his metal wristwatch because it became too loose; he noticed this when the tan line around his watch began to show—it was the tan line that caught his eye.
- A 39-year-old reported being able to pull the airplane tray table down without hitting his stomach.

My professional and personal passions united in my practice. I could now blend the pleasure of writing recipes on prescription slips with the chance to empower motivated people to transform their lives.

As I continued work in my practice, I began to see a pattern emerge—it was mostly men who were coming to me, and they were achieving knockout, sustained results.

I knew this was a statistical anomaly. Men notoriously shy away from "diets" and balk at traditional dieting rules. Counting points or calories, eating smaller portions, and consuming low-fat, low-sugar, low-flavor versions of everything aren't concepts that bring most men to the table. But something about my approach was not only bringing them to the table, it was helping them embrace this gut-free, pain-free, ready-for-action solution. And sometimes, they got to leave behind the pill bottles they no longer needed.

> **HOT TIP**
>
> Losing just 10 pounds can lower your blood pressure. Track your pressure at home and show your doctor the numbers. Decide together whether you can adjust your medication.

REFUEL EMERGES

In writing this book, I went back and re-read and analyzed the file of every man I've treated over the last fifteen years, paying attention to what worked for each and what didn't. I analyzed thousands of peer-reviewed clinical reports in metabolism and endocrinology to find the science behind the most successful strategies. I read all of the comments on my *ChefMD*® and *Paging Dr. La Puma* blogs and the recipe postings from over 30,000 subscribers. (Join them! Sign up at www .drjohnlapuma.com for tools and advice.)

After all that research, one fact struck me immediately: there is no such thing as a unisex diet. If a man wants to lose weight, a diet designed to help women will not usually work.

When it comes to the subject of weight, men and women couldn't be more different. Not only do men feel differently about food, we metabolize it differently, carry our weight differently, store our fat differently, and burn fat differently and at different rates with exercise. We have completely different attitudes toward and expectations of weight-control programs.

> **MAN MEMO**
>
> Men who went to exclusively male weight-loss meetings lost twice as much weight as those who attended co-ed meetings.

These differences are obvious when you look at many current diet books and programs. Nearly all popular diets and diet books have been written for women. Almost no programs have been created just for men to meet their distinct medical, physiological, and behavioral needs. That is, until now.

> ## MAN MEMO
> Men generally have greater muscle mass and lower body fat than women. More muscle and less fat means men need 10 to 15 percent more calories than their female counterparts to maintain their weight.

What you're looking at in this book is a scientifically sound and clinically proven weight-loss and weight-maintenance program designed specifically for *men*. It makes guys feel better, right away. It shows them how to ratchet their efforts up to the next level, without cutting out whole food groups as fad diets do, and without getting overwhelmed by a lot of the science that is not all that relevant to the subject at hand.

The program sticks to the science you actually *need* to keep you on track, to catch you if you fall, and to let your body work efficiently so you can lose the gut. The program is also about self-improvement: it allows your inherent but occasionally dormant confidence in yourself and your life purpose to re-emerge.

Before I dive into the details of the program, let's rewind for a quick macro view of men's health today. You will see, if you don't already do so when you look in the mirror, why it's more important than ever that you reprogram your body and recharge your life.

THE EPIDEMIC OF THE MID-WAIST CRISIS

Throughout the United States, nearly three out of four men are at an unhealthy weight. In fact, there are more overweight and obese men in every state than there are overweight and obese women. The numbers not only travel across state lines but also across ethnicities; only Asian and Pacific Islander men have overweight numbers below 50 percent—and even then, 42 percent of them are overweight or obese. Across the board, men are quite literally being weighed down by their weight, and they are paying the price of lost strength, stamina, and energy.

Even more concerning is where the excess fat tissue shows up on a man: the gut. And that's when a major genetic disadvantage emerges. The type of weight gain that men experience gives them the "gut" or beer belly, and earns them the nickname of "Santa" or "Buddha" or "Big." This situation has contributed to what I refer to as the "mid-waist crisis" that millions of men are experiencing today. Worse than a mid-life crisis, the mid-waist crisis can attack your body from the inside and bring you down—as deep as six feet under.

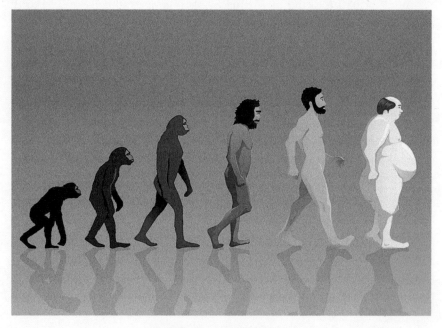

The Evolution: A Mid-Waist Crisis

In 2008, researchers came to a frightening conclusion after monitoring nearly 360,000 men and women for ten years: increased abdominal fat had doubled their risk of premature death. To those of us in the medical field, this study confirmed a theory that had been developing for decades. To the general public, it scientifically defined a new public health enemy: belly fat.

▶ HOW MUCH IS TOO MUCH?

More than total weight or body mass index (BMI), your waist circumference is the simplest and most efficient gauge of your metabolic and hormonal health. Here are three methods I suggest my patients use for measuring belly fat:

1. Take a tape measure and wrap it around your bare-skin abdominal region right at your belly button. Check the number. What is it? Anything over 40 inches is too much. (For a woman, 35 inches or less is the goal.)
2. Stand naked in front of a full-length mirror. Turn sideways and look at yourself in the mirror. For men, which is farther out—your stomach or your penis? If it's your stomach, it's too big.
3. Still naked and standing, tilt your head back and look at the ceiling. Now, bring your head forward and put your chin on your chest. See anything below your belly? You should. If you don't, there's a problem. (In other words, #cycyp—can you see your penis?)

Belly fat, also known as intra-abdominal fat and scientifically referred to as visceral fat, is more than just an unattractive gathering of fat cells covering your abs. It is an insidious, metabolically active type of fat that deposits inside and around your organs. It's more than just unappealing to the eye—it can be deadly. Once entrenched there, visceral fat spews out hormones and toxins that disrupt your natural biological functions.

While its first course of action may be to ding your self-confidence, visceral fat goes on to do much greater damage inside your body. Admit it: when your stomach has prevented you from giving a full embrace to an attractive individual, you may have sucked in your gut or hugged the air, Hollywood style.

This type of fat has also been linked to an ever-growing list of metabolic disturbances and diseases, including diabetes, endothelial dysfunction (a rusting on the inside of your arteries and a precursor to heart disease), erectile dysfunction, heart disease, high cholesterol, hypertension, insulin resistance, and colon cancer. As one researcher claimed, "Visceral obesity does seem to be truly evil."

Men gain this dangerous type of fat first, whereas women are more inclined to gain subcutaneous fat tissue—the squishy, pinchable type of fat. Visceral fat is dense and firm to the touch. No, that's not muscle pushing your stomach out beyond your pants; it's packed-in visceral fat.

> **MAN MEMO**
> Women can gain up to 44 more pounds of body fat than men, on average, before they experience the same severity of risk factors.

The *Journal of Clinical Investigation* published a study evaluating each gender's metabolic risk profile at the same level of body fat. Men had higher total cholesterol, triglycerides, and blood sugar than did women, and lower levels of high-density lipoprotein (HDL)—what's considered to be the "good" or "healthy" cholesterol. Talk about being set up for failure. But wait, the plot—not just your blood—thickens.

When the researchers sat these men and women down for a meal and then measured their metabolic responses, men continued to be worse off: they showed higher levels of triglycerides and lagged behind in ability to clear out the triglycerides quickly. Triglycerides are a form of troublemaker fat in your blood—like teenagers drinking beer in front of your house, you don't want them loitering around. Chronically elevated triglycerides have been linked to coronary artery disease, a condition significantly more prevalent in men, and to small, beady, dense, damaging LDL cholesterol.

Visceral fat was to blame for these stubborn triglycerides, and labeled the "best predictor" of the delayed ability to clear out fats from the blood. The study left little room for doubt: men have more visceral fat and it doesn't just sit idly by. It gets involved, and not with good intentions.

Visceral fat likes to nestle itself around several important organs and settle close to the portal vein, which drains from the small intestine into the liver. What researchers have found is that visceral fat will dump inflammatory proteins and hormones into the portal vein, sending them directly down to the liver. That is, visceral fat is your polluting neighbor who dumps paint thinner and motor oil on the ground . . . to leach into your water supply.

YOUR CHOLESTEROL SCORE

High cholesterol can be a leading indicator of serious health risks like athero-sclerosis, or hardening of the arteries. If you haven't had your cholesterol levels checked in the last year and you are over the age of 40, I strongly encourage you to do so. At-home kits are now being offered for convenience and for the doctor averse—they're not quite as perfect as a formal, laboratory examination of fluids, but they can give you a pretty good gauge of where you stand.

Ultimately, tests that measure particle size can tell you how much of the most dangerous type of cholesterol you have in your blood. The small and dense type of LDL cholesterol is beady and penetrates your arteries; the large and fluffy forms of LDL are not as bad. But tests that measure particle size and pattern are often expensive, hard to obtain, and hard to interpret. The real goal of cholesterol screening is to predict cardiac risk, which can be done by keeping an eye on your overall levels.

Here's how to read your basic test results:

TOTAL CHOLESTEROL

Below 200 mg/dL is ideal
200–239 mg/dL is borderline high
240 mg/dL is high

LDL CHOLESTEROL

Below 100 mg/dL is ideal
100–129 mg/dL is a safe range
130–159 mg/dL is borderline high
Over 160 mg/dL is high
Over 190 mg/dL is very high

HDL CHOLESTEROL

Over 50 mg/dL is good
Over 60 mg/dL is even better

TRIGLYCERIDES

Below 150 mg/dL is recommended

Source: The American Heart Association, September 2013

> **MAN MEMO**
> The term "viscera" is used to describe the organs located inside your abdominal cavity. The liver, stomach, small intestines, and others all fit into place there like a brilliantly designed puzzle. That is, until interloper visceral fat works itself deviously into the mix.

The liver does its best to filter out any toxins before sending blood back out to your body for use, but it can process only so much at a time. Too much visceral fat means an overabundance of inflammatory substances, leading to chronic inflammation—a condition that's been connected to diabetes, cancer, depression, stroke, Alzheimer's, and heart disease.

Whether by way of chronic inflammation or other metabolic disturbances, being overweight independently increases your chances of developing twenty different kinds of cancer—in fact, obesity has surpassed tobacco smoking as the leading cause of cancer. In men, the strongest associations occur with cancer of the esophagus, kidney, pancreas, and colon—the last of which is connected specifically to increased waist circumference. And U.S. men have nearly 20 percent more invasive cancer than do women: more colon cancer, more rectal cancer, more lung and bronchial cancer.

What does all this boil down to for you? It means that as a man you have a biological disadvantage when it comes to weight gain. You gain the most dangerous type of fat first, and this sets you up for a battery of health issues, beginning with seemingly manageable conditions like high blood pressure and high cholesterol, spiraling into more serious conditions such as heart disease, fatty liver, and type-2 diabetes, and ending in an increased risk for premature death and disability. Fortunately, while you might have some cards stacked against you, there is still hope.

The good news is there's a way to avoid and even reverse this process. Just because you are a man doesn't mean you have to follow this path. In fact, *because* you are a man, you can overcome it with a smart, strategic plan that reprograms your body from the very physiological source of your manhood: testosterone (which you'll see referred to as "T" throughout the book). It turns out that the same vital sex hormone that's been steering so many of your biological functions since puberty can play a crucial role in the regulation of visceral fat and the severity of its effects.

> **MAN MEMO**
> Testosterone (T) exposure in the womb has been linked to determination of facial shape and physical ability. There's no going back to build a stronger jawline, but you can boost your strength, as Refueled men have done in just 24 days, with increased T-levels. (#tboost)

Belly Fat and Your Metabolic Functions

Metabolically speaking, men and women are quite different. The most prominent difference lies in the sex hormones, testosterone and estrogen. Men have much higher levels of the androgen testosterone, which is synthesized in the testes from cholesterol, while women have more estrogen, which is produced by the ovaries and fat tissue.

From a health standpoint, it's desirable for you to have a little bit of estrogen in your body, but here "little" is the key word: elevated levels of estrogen in men have been connected to increased risk of stroke, heart disease, and prostate cancer. Research has shown that often when increased estrogen is present, so too is abdominal obesity.

> **MAN MEMO**
> Testosterone and estrogen are moved throughout your body by a transporter known as sex hormone–binding globulin (SHBG). This protein also helps prevent T and estrogen from degrading and trying to leave the body.

The snap judgment would be that the fat is entirely to blame. We already know that visceral fat is the bad guy, and it's just as guilty when it comes to messing with your sex hormones. But visceral fat doesn't create all this chaos on its own; it produces aromatase, the enzyme that does all the damage. When aromatase is present, it takes free-floating testosterone and converts it to estrogen—an irreversible conversion that can have disastrous effects on men. This type of hormonal imbalance shrinks a man's testes, softens his skin, erodes his beard, enlarges his breasts, dampens his sex drive, and weakens his erections.

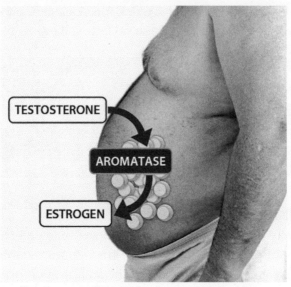

Testosterone-to-Estrogen Conversion: How It Happens

Source: www.drjohnlapuma.com

As this imbalance continues, it further programs the body to store more belly fat. The more fat stored, the more aromatase, the less testosterone, and the more estrogen—the cycle is set. As visceral fat accumulation rises, so too do the biological dysfunctions. Greater visceral fat leads to insulin and leptin resistance, which in turn leads to further weight gain and a high triglyceride/low HDL pattern, which spirals into greater risk for heart disease, stroke, erectile dysfunction, pre-diabetes, and type-2 diabetes.

THE INSULIN CONNECTION

Insulin is one of the most important hormones your body produces. Your pancreas makes insulin when foods have been broken down into glucose and the glucose is ready to be moved into cells and tissues for use. Insulin transports this usable energy to the appropriate cells and, once there, acts as a key to "unlock" your cells so they can take in the critical fuel. Insulin also decides when you should store fuel as fat and when you need to use it for energy. Bottom line: you don't want anything to get in insulin's way. Now, guess what goes out of its way to get into insulin's way? Visceral fat, of course.

Visceral fat reduces insulin sensitivity and promotes insulin resistance, which are both well-known precursors to diabetes. Belly fat drives up the inflammatory proteins known as cytokines, which when constantly produced lead to chronic inflammation. And, once your body hits this inflammatory state, it will most likely lose insulin sensitivity. Your pancreas will keep producing insulin, but your cells essentially become numb to it. You've then hit full-blown insulin resistance. Prolonged insulin resistance can lead to diabetes, high blood pressure, arteriosclerosis, and heart disease.

Food is the key: men who eat to lose the gut also improve their insulin sensitivity, increase their testosterone levels naturally, and get leaner where it counts—in the waist.

When you add the natural effects of age to this equation—specifically, increasing body fat and decreasing muscle beginning in middle age—it would seem that men's bodies are destined to fail them. But before you toss in the towel, let me tell you that this equation for certain destruction leaves out one tiny element on which all these biological and metabolic mechanisms rely—food.

What you eat is directly responsible for how your body functions and forms, from the ground floor on up. Food triggers hormone release, directs fat distribution, choreographs cellular and mitochondrial performance, and changes the proteins your genes make. Food really is the source of power.

▶ AROMATASE ON OVERDRIVE

A study published in the journal *Molecular and Cellular Endocrinology* concluded that the consumption of poor-quality carbs increased the activity of aromatase, which "TURBOCHARGE[D]" the production of estrogen, accelerated fat storage, and promoted metabolic syndrome, type-2 diabetes, and prostate cancer. (I've maintained the capital letters from the original study—the authors clearly wanted to leave little room for doubt.) Minimizing your consumption of highly processed carbohydrates will drastically curtail the production of aromatase and help keep your testosterone intact.

So, extend this to say that you've been eating what's been fed to you by the dominant food culture (i.e., highly processed food products, not real foods). And it has worsened the problem of visceral fat and the cascade of health issues that come with it. The simple solution should be to eat differently. In fact, eating differently *is* the solution, but there has to be more to it than that; you have to become mindful of the male biology. Which is why traditional dieting will not help you.

Let's take a look at why traditional dieting might have led you right back to where you started—or failed to entice you to start at all.

WE HAVE SYSTEMS FAILURE

Nutritionists have failed men in weight control because they have neglected the importance of strategy and instead have focused on calories, carbs, fat, and protein. Nutritionists have not focused on looking and feeling better, getting lean and strong, avoiding future health problems, and losing the gut. Nutritionists also have not focused on how men gain weight and why, nor have they created a program that starts with men in mind.

Medicine has had little research on men and weight control. Even something as important as aromatase was overlooked for years in men's health because excess estrogen was presumed to be relevant only to women.

Without a doubt, there have been plenty of health and fitness books written for men, but they're mostly written for the *one guy*—the one who is already obviously fit or balances right on the edge; the one who just wants to "pack on a little extra muscle"; the one whose jeans size hasn't changed in ten years; the one who eats as much pizza as you do but never has a grease stain on his shirt or a spare tire to show for it. The *one guy* hits the gym, is always eating miniature granola bars, runs and cycles, and may even brag about his "awesome workout last night at yoga." If you don't know this guy personally, you know him from Photoshopped magazine articles and infomercials. Let's refer to this *one guy* as "the guy who doesn't need this book."

You are probably not that guy—most of us aren't. What if, like my patient Brad, you're looking just to take it up a step or two? Up until now you've had few options other than to turn to the overwhelming number of diet books written for women.

It doesn't help men that most have been in denial about their weight and the health risks it presents, despite the fact that excess weight is more dangerous to men than to women. Unfortunately, this head-in-the-sand response to health issues doesn't bode well for quality of life or longevity—men are likely to die on average five years earlier than women.

> **MAN MEMO**
> Do you have an accurate gauge of your weight? Here's one: no scale required. Your waist circumference should be half your height in inches. Any higher, and it's time to drop some belly fat.

As a medical professional and a man, it gives me hope to be able to say that I've seen firsthand how the attitude toward manly weight loss is changing. When my male patients begin their programs, they ordinarily don't believe it will work. Because nothing else ever has.

They figure they'll just wind up eating the high-fat, high-sugar foods that they eat anyway, because they're discouraged or because the foods are handy. These men think they will be stuck forever taking their medications for back pain or depression or diabetes or cholesterol or blood pressure. They'll continue to carry the same risk of heart disease as their dad or their brother or their uncle has. Or had.

But then something happens. Their belt buckles move one hole over—in the right direction. Their wives or girlfriends start picking out new clothes for them. Their wristwatches get looser and slide a little bit around their wrists. They feel better. A lot better.

They ultimately discover that Refuel isn't like everything else they've tried, or even thought about trying. They discover that I haven't taken a cookie-cutter approach to helping them lose their gut. That I know if a man wants to lose weight, a diet designed to help a woman will not work. That there are specific and strategic reasons Refuel works for men.

Let me tell you a little more about it.

A MAN, A PLAN

Refuel is an eating and lifestyle plan that is designed to suit your preferences for food and exercise, and to play to your natural habits and rituals. I'll bet you want better health, but you don't want to go to a lot of meetings (or maybe even read a whole book) to achieve it. I'll bet you want to eat better than a can of chunky beef stew. I'll bet you're interested in flavor, but less interested in an ingredient list of twenty-five items. I believe you are more adventurous with food than people give you credit for, but that often you just want a simple meal that's satisfying. I'm pretty sure you think you don't like to exercise hard—or you really don't because it causes you pain and discomfort—but you also really want to feel and be strong.

> **▶ HOT TIP**
>
> Go easy on your joints: 1 pound of weight loss can take up to 4 pounds of pressure off your knees.

What happens when you follow an eating plan written specifically for your body type and biology—one that's designed to help you feel what life is like without a gut that's too big? A great and profound change occurs in your life.

A reprogramming takes place—not overnight, but in less time than you think. One morning you wake up in a body that you don't have to drag out of bed; that gives you energy to tackle the day, not shrink from it; that makes movement pleasurable, not painful; that brings back to life the competitive edge in you, so you can hear the voice inside your head that pushes you to go further and harder, at work, on the golf course or at the gym, and in the bedroom. You wake up feeling like a man more in control of his own life.

To get serious, you must get organized (I show you how). You make the healthy options be your automatic, default options (I show you how). You have to take care of business and remodel your environment, little by little. (I will show you how, but you have to put in the work. I didn't say this was crazy easy. I said it worked.)

And once you've succeeded—and you will succeed—you work on keeping what you've achieved. You create a metabolic motor. You regenerate muscle tissue and generate more mitochondria, the power plants in your cells. You make them do the work. You become your healthy lifestyle. You feel the payback personally, and it feels really, really good.

I've laid out this book to get you quick, clear, and accurate nuggets of gold (#nog™)—crucial, actionable information you need to change your body and your life, starting today. I offer Man Memos, Hot Tips, Fast Stats, and Chef's Secrets to clue you in, right away. I'll show you how to master the essential male trifecta of exercise, sleep, and mindset/stress management. I'll show you how to identify the most time-efficient bursts of cardio and muscle-building resistance exercises, so your body begins to do the work for you, safely. I'll show you how to build growth hormone, critical for muscle tissue growth and fat burning, and to build testosterone as you sleep. I'll show you how to make stress productive instead of frustrating, so you respond instead of react. You'll revise your mindset and reset your endocrine system in your favor, so that you burn the calories in your bloodstream instead of storing them as fat.

> ## MAN MEMO
> It may be only the size of a pea, but the pituitary gland is a big deal for men: it's responsible for sending out luteinizing hormone (LH), which signals the testes to make more testosterone.

You'll find these strategies and their supporting science throughout the book. Once we get to Part Three, I'll direct you through the program, where you'll discover five commandments and three distinct phases. Here is a preview.

REFUEL PHASES

Phase 1: *Jumpstart* = 3 days

In this phase, you'll eat to accelerate visceral fat loss and regulate your metabolic response to foods. We focus on keeping carbohydrates to no more than 50 grams a day for three days. Later, we do just two consecutive days of up to 50 grams of carbs each day. Most processed carbs don't keep you full for long and they promote excessive insulin response, leading to increased belly-fat storage and decreased energy. The carbohydrates you eat will come from fruits, vegetables, whole grains, dairy, legumes, and nuts. You'll eat foods with more protein because these foods will make it easier to form lean muscle tissue and keep you fuller longer. And you'll eat foods with healthy fats: they do not spike insulin.

Phase 2: *Boost Growth Hormone and Testosterone* = 14 days

For each week of this two-week phase, you will apply Phase 1 guidelines for two consecutive days. On the other five days of each week, you will eat vegetables and foods rich in lean proteins, and smaller amounts of whole grains, tree nuts, fruit, and full-fat dairy. You will also implement my strategy for minimizing your daily exposure to the toxins and chemical pollutants that are increasingly being linked to metabolic disturbances, specifically to reduced levels of testosterone and related increases in estrogen and estrogen-like hormones in men. The next chapter will delve deeply into the scary, persuasive links among toxins, obesity, and hormones.

Phase 3: *Maximize Energy* = 7 days

For two of the seven days in this phase, you will stick to the same plan as Phase 1. On the other five days, you'll work on strengthening your skills using the master goals. With enough practice they will become a permanent part of your life. You will also add in a splurge meal, if you want, one day per week. Eat anything you want for that meal—only. Then, it's back on plan. Since this is designed to be a phase that you can transition into as your long-term way of eating, I'll teach you how to study food labels and learn to read them better, how to sensibly enjoy wine or beer with meals, and how to further expand your palate for more adventurous eating. This phase, you stay on for good.

To get a Refuel Cheat Sheet highlighting what you need to do during each phase and to score other free book bonuses, visit www.drjohnlapuma .com.

THE COMPLETE PACKAGE

Each phase of Refuel will be accompanied by sample menu plans and instructions for which foods to eat and recipes to try out. In just 24 days, you will have learned the essentials of preparing delicious meals at home, as well as how to find or make healthy, filling meal alternatives when you are traveling. You'll emerge with five essential cooking methods that you'll have for life, and enjoy fifteen man-tested essential recipes that will keep you satisfied, and will surprise and impress your family and friends. When you're ready to add to your arsenal, visit www.drjohnlapuma.com.

CHEF'S SECRET

Are you man enough to master the "fundamental five"?

1. Blend
2. Simmer
3. Grill
4. Roast
5. Stir-fry

Put your skills to the test in Chapter 12.

The three phases will also integrate the weapons-trifecta men have available in addition to diet: sleep, exercise, and stress optimization. It's easy to push these areas of your life under the rug or let them go on as they may. The problem is, when these aspects of your life are ignored, they will slowly unravel your health until you're an out-of-breath time bomb with high blood pressure who doubles as a sleep-deprived zombie with excess belly fat.

MAN MEMO

"If you cannot measure it, you cannot improve it," said physicist Lord Kelvin. So, measure we will. In Chapter 4, you'll find three quizzes: (1) to test your T level, (2) to check in on your habits, and (3) to help you create goals. Measure first; improvement will follow.

The first step is to just start paying attention and self-track: How much sleep do you get? How little exercise? How do you respond to stress? The answers might clue you in to ways to make easy, small changes to feel at your best.

I'm going to teach you how to get your best back. By applying my Rest, Exercise, and Unwind protocol (RE-UP), you'll maximize weight loss and boost energy levels. Each phase of the Refuel program will include a RE-UP section in which I provide quick, simple strategies for sleeping better, exercising smarter, and retooling your mindset, so you can perform your best, even when there is chronic stress. Read, and then apply to your daily life.

IT'S YOUR TURN

Every guy I know has a to-do list. Put yourself on that to-do list. Start this program tomorrow. Remember to visit www.drjohnlapuma.com, where you can sign up for my newsletter and get free book bonuses to help you on your way. There's no shame in weight gain, but there is no courage in not trying to be healthier, better, and stronger than you are now. Don't push the delete button when you see a photo you don't like. Because changing it is within your power—without Photoshop.

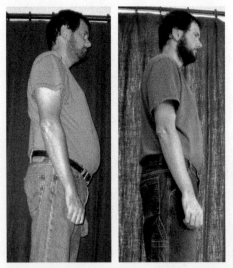

Day I   Day 24

REFUEL SUCCESS
Name: **Owen B.**
Age: **34**
Weight Loss in 24 Days: **20 pounds**
Waist Loss: **3 inches**

The Weight Gain

During three years spent in Africa as a volunteer math and science teacher, Owen B. never thought much about weight: "I was constantly active and I got ill—not the best weight-loss plan, but I was definitely thin."

It wasn't until Owen and his wife moved to New Mexico that he picked up the American (he's Welsh) habits of eating out all the time and drinking lots of soda. "When we ate at home we were good, but eating out wasn't helpful—I definitely ate a lot of fries."

Despite being fairly active, Owen found himself at a personal all-time-high weight of 220 pounds. Yet he wanted to keep up with his two young children, to be an active dad and husband. "I was ready to be healthy for myself and for my family. I wanted to have fewer aches and pains and to just feel fitter overall."

What Changed

Owen had started making small changes and noticed some weight loss, but it had stalled; he was hoping to avoid the slow drift back up to his higher weight.

He knew he wanted to stick to Refuel pretty strictly, so he turned to technology; as a Web developer he was already using apps and programs to help manage daily life. For tracking what he ate, Owen relied on an app from myfitnesspal.com. "This allowed me to log foods and scan barcodes so items were automatically entered in," says Owen. "The first couple of days on the plan I was at a work conference so it was trial by fire—but logging everything helped me make sure I was on track, especially on the 50 grams of carbs days."

After two weeks of being meticulous about monitoring and educating himself on food values, Owen felt he had learned enough to let his new knowledge do a lot of the work. "I had a good sense of what I should be eating by then."

As a vegetarian, he made sure to get enough protein from foods like eggs and tofu. Here's what an average day looked like for him:

BREAKFAST: Hard-boiled or fried eggs with a veggie sausage patty
or a smoothie with protein powder and coconut milk
or a big bowl of steamed vegetables

LUNCH:	Huge salad with a veggie burger and some grilled vegetables
	or a quick heat-and-eat meal like Thai coconut soup
DINNER:	Tofu or seitan and vegetable stir-fry
	or veggie omelet and roasted vegetables

Exercise was monitored with a tracking tool, too: "I found an app on my phone called Impetus that allowed me to program intervals into it so I didn't have to think during workouts—the timer let me know when I was done."

He also looked for ways to work more activity into his days. "I started riding my bike down to the beach to check out the ocean, and I began using an indoor climbing wall. I didn't want to just run on a treadmill—these types of activities were more enjoyable and also happened to make me more active."

What's Better Now

"Overall I just feel more confident. My trousers fit now and I actually need to go out and buy new ones," says Owen. "And I'm stronger—I feel my muscles engage more even with everyday movements."

It's not just his family who has noticed the weight loss. "I went to the farmers' market and had people there ask me if I'd lost weight, people I know only casually—it feels good."

Best Tips

- **Use the Refuel Commandments.** "I really followed the guideline to not eat things I can crush, which worked great for me. I focused instead on loading up on vegetables and getting more of them when I could, like adding spinach to my smoothies. It really does fill you up."
- **Incorporate more movement throughout your day.** "I work from home and use a stand-up desk, but just standing can get uncomfortable. I bought a treadmill on Craigslist and now walk on that as I work. It improved my work environment and helped me add in multiple miles of walking to each day."
- **Track religiously, at least at first.** "That was key for me—it made it so I didn't have to think too much."

2

TOXINS

They'll Kill You, but First They'll Make You Fat

We live in dangerous times. While significantly less dangerous than, say, the Dark Ages, when plague was lurking around every bend, our current environment is not without its perils. Consider these headlines, for example:

- *Canada, 30 U.S. States Affected by Ground Beef, Other Cuts Recalled Due to E. Coli Contamination (Oct. 2012)*
- *Over 240 Brands Recall Peanut-Based Products That May Have Been Tainted with Salmonella (Sept. 2012)*
- *114 Tons of Spinach Recalled After Traces of E. Coli Bacteria Detected (Dec. 2011)*
- *65 Rice Products Found to Contain Arsenic (Sept. 2012)*

Listeria, E. coli, and salmonella are all examples of pathogenic bacteria that carry and cause disease. Their risks are well known, which is why foods from farms and factories are routinely sampled and tested by the FDA (clearly, their system is not without its flaws). Most often a person who consumes bacteria-laden food makes a full recovery on his or her own, sometimes after a short bout of unadulterated misery.

But what if I told you there were worse things entering your body every single moment of every single day? That there are invisible toxins and chemical additives flowing into your body from all directions? They are found in the water you drink, the foods you eat (even the organic ones), the pills you take, the air you breathe, and the clothes you wear. The problem with many of these toxins and chemical additives is that they don't signal your body to purge itself of a harmful invader. They instead slip past your body's filters undetected, and once inside begin to disrupt functions critical to testosterone and growth-hormone synthesis, metabolism, and reproductive health.

Avoiding all toxins, additives, and heavy metals these days is impossible, but in this chapter you'll learn about the worst offenders and get some practical applications for reducing your own personal chemical intake. Chances are that right now, it's off the charts.

> **MAN MEMO**

Keep your consumption of these mercury-ridden fish low and you'll avoid the fatigue, nausea, headaches, and tremors that can accompany mercury toxicity:

Mackerel (King)
Marlin
Orange roughy
Shark
Swordfish
Tilefish
Tuna (Bigeye, Ahi)

I'll also identify in this chapter the common prescription medicines that cause stealth weight gain. In many cases, losing the fat and building a harder body can reduce the need for these medicines.

By diminishing your exposure to the chemicals that drop testosterone levels and retard muscle growth, you can use your metabolic advantages to control your weight and improve your general health.

> **HOT TIP**
> Mitochondria are the powerhouses of your cells, fulfilling 90 percent of your body's energy needs. Fuel them properly and you'll turn up the fat burning and increase your energy. Eat more magnesium-rich foods; halibut, cooked spinach, and pumpkin seeds are top sources. Try Pan-Seared Mahimahi with Red Cabbage (p. 217) to give yourself some high-octane mitochondrial fuel packed with flavor.

THE ERA OF OVEREXPOSURE

In 2010, the President's Cancer Panel of the National Institutes of Health (NIH) issued a report on the prevalence of environmental risks in which they revealed that 80,000 or more chemicals are currently in use in the United States. The frightening part: only a few hundred of the 80,000 have been tested for safety.

Of that long list of chemicals, there are a select few that have proved to be a specific and serious threat to men's health. Of course, many others could prove even more dangerous down the road, but the research in this area has only recently begun to hit its stride. There are some xenoestrogens, antiandrogens, and persistent organic pollutants. (Don't worry—there won't be a spelling test at the end.)

GENDER BENDERS

For men, of particular concern are xenoestrogens and antiandrogens. Xenoestrogens are foreign estrogens that come from pesticides, chemicals, herbicides, food additives, food containers, and detergents. These impostor hormones can be more powerful than the body's own, strong enough to counteract your testosterone and create significant hormonal imbalance. Antiandrogens block testosterone and dihydrotestosterone (DHT) from bonding to an androgen receptor, thereby interfering with sperm production, libido, erections, hair growth, muscle development, and basically every other secondary sexual characteristic that makes you a man.

By mimicking or blocking important sex hormones you make, xenoestrogens or antiandrogens lead to dramatically out-of-balance hormones. When your estrogen and testosterone levels are out of balance you don't build muscle or burn fat efficiently, your skin is too smooth, you have man boobs ("moobs") or love handles, and you have trouble getting it up. Essentially, you begin to turn into a girl (#turnyouintoa girl).

Both xenoestrogens and antiandrogens are endocrine disrupters. They can prevent natural biological functions and force unnatural modifications. Hormones that were intended to be eliminated by the body get stuck there; others that were meant to make connections don't make them; critical feedback loops break down. When these disruptions continue, weaknesses develop and diseases follow. In men, endocrine disrupters have been linked to erectile dysfunction, infertility, testicular and prostate cancers, immune suppression, and malfunctions in the pituitary glands.

> **MAN MEMO**
> Your body has two main systems of communication: the nervous system and the endocrine system. The first works like 4G, sending rapid-delivery messages via the neurons. The second usually operates more like a dial-up connection, with glands and organs sending out messenger hormones by way of the bloodstream.

Let's look at a few of the worst of these hormonal evil-doers and how they could be affecting your health.

Bisphenol-A

A chemical compound found in polycarbonate plastics and epoxy resins, Bisphenol-A (aka BPA) is used in all sorts of plastic goods, including water bottles, food packaging, sunglasses, and medical devices. As a resin, it is employed to line canned goods and can also be used as a dental sealant. Another common use of BPA is in receipts and tickets—any kind of "thermal" printing on a receipt or ticket, say from a gas station, movie, or travel, has extremely high levels of BPA.

In 2008, BPA became a "celebrity toxin," for its bad behavior. By that time, hundreds of studies had been done and many of them connected BPA to reproductive problems, increased levels of prostate and breast cancer, cardiovascular issues, and impaired fetal development.

In fact, BPA hit men where it hurts. In the *Journal of Andrology* (andrology is the study of men, especially fertility and sexual function), researchers determined that high levels of BPA were strongly correlated with declining sexual function. Men with high BPA levels in their urine reported "decreased sexual desire, more difficulty having an erection, lower ejaculation strength, and lower level of overall satisfaction with sex life." The blame was placed on BPA's estrogenic and antiandrogenic effects.

Other recent studies have shown the dangers of BPA exposure in all humans. Scientists publishing in the *Journal of the American Medical Association* reported that individuals with high levels of BPA were twice as likely to have diabetes or heart disease.

Finally, some people are paying attention to the research and are phasing BPA out of certain products. In 2012, the FDA banned BPA from use in baby bottles and kids' "sippy" cups. And standard brands like Campbell's soups have declared they would stop using BPA to line their cans. This is especially good news, since studies have shown that canned soup consumption can increase the amount of BPA in the urine by 1,000 percent. Many popular stainless-steel bottle makers have also stopped using BPA to line their products.

▶ GO AWAY BPA

Watch out for acidic items in metal containers; high-acid foods such as sodas, citrus, and tomatoes can induce greater breakdown of BPA in container linings. Some brands, such as Muir Glen, Eden Organic, and Trader Joe's, are now packaging foods in BPA-free containers.

I think we're just beginning to see the real potential damage this ubiquitous substance can cause, which is why the more proactive you can be in avoiding it, the better.

What You Can Do

- **Skip the receipt.** A lot of companies are now offering to email or text you your sales receipt; if you are ever given that option, jump at the chance. In 2010, researchers found that thermal receipts from stores like CVS, Safeway, and Whole Foods had high levels of BPA. The BPA on these receipts and other thermal-coated papers easily transfers to your hands and is tough to remove even with a good hand washing. If you touch any mucous membrane, such as by sampling a sauce on your finger or picking your nose, you transfer that BPA straight to your bloodstream. If you need to keep your sales receipts, drop them into an envelope or your wallet, not into your pocket.
- **Stay clear of #7 (most of the time).** The majority of plastic packaging has a number stamped on the bottom, indicating what types of compounds were used in its production. Plastics marked with #7 are the most likely to contain BPA, but some can be labeled "BPA-Free," so look for this text on the packaging. Better options are plastics marked with #2, #4, and #5.

 If you see this unlucky #7 on plastic packaging and no "BPA-Free" text appears on the label, put the item back.

- **Avoid heating plastics.** Even though the sturdier plastic containers can withstand the heat of a microwave oven or the hot water in a dishwasher, don't subject them to high heat, including extended exposure to the sun. If a BPA-containing plastic is heated, it will release even more of the compound into the food or beverage it is holding, is wrapped around, or is stuck to.
- **Use more stainless steel, ceramic, or glass containers.** Try to drink only filtered water from a BPA-free stainless-steel, ceramic, or glass bottle. Store your foods and beverages in containers made from these materials as much as possible.

> **HOT TIP**

There are plenty of companies now making BPA-free reusable plastic bottles. For everyday use, however, try nonplastic containers—at least when you're at home. Here are some manufacturers and their websites:

Glass	Stainless Steel
Takeya: http://www.takeyausa.com/	SIGG: http://www.mysigg.com/
Lifefactory: http://www.lifefactory.com/	Kleen Kanteen: http://www.kleankanteen.com/
Pure: http://pureglassbottle.com/	Alex: http://www.alexbottle.com/

- Opt for fresh or frozen or jarred instead of canned foods. Even though companies like Campbell's are making an effort to remove the BPA from their packaging, the compound is still not banned, so eating fresh, frozen, or jarred foods is the safer option.

PHTHALATES

Added to plastics, phthalates (pronounced THAL-ates) make them more flexible. You'll find them in children's toys, garden hoses, food packaging, toothbrushes, tools, shower curtains, and vinyl flooring. Phthalates are also used in a lot of liquid products with a fragrance because they help extend the life of the fragrance.

These compounds, which are often referred to as "plasticizers," are everywhere. They're also *in* just about everyone around you. The CDC's *National Report on Human Exposure to Environmental*

Chemicals, published in 2009, noted that nearly 80 percent of the population had evidence of phthalates in their urine.

> ## MAN MEMO
> Researchers found that three days of eating foods free of plastics lowered the BPA levels in people's urine by two-thirds; phthalate levels dropped by more than half.

Phthalates are especially dangerous to us because they don't bond permanently to whatever plastic into which they have been mixed. That means that when the plastic ages or is heated, the phthalates are easily released into whatever else is around. That could be your food, the air, your skin, or your toddler's mouth when he starts gnawing on those plastic blocks. And, of course, this process of transfer is invisible to the human eye. There's no yelling, "Wait! Get that phthalate out of your mouth!"

So, why are the phthalates a problem for guys? Because they're a bona fide antiandrogen, and so they will fight against everything that's male about you—from the very beginning of your life. Prenatal exposure to high levels of phthalates has been connected to delayed genital development in boys ages 2 to 36 months. It doesn't get much better when you're older, either: phthalates inhibit testosterone production in adult men, contribute to a declining sperm count, and cause DNA damage to the sperm.

Also, the disruption doesn't stop with the reproductive issues. In 2007, a group of researchers hypothesized that if phthalates were lowering the testosterone in males, then they were also contributing to the increases in abdominal obesity and insulin resistance. (Remember: optimal hormone levels often correlate to healthy body weight.) Sure enough, their research revealed that higher phthalate levels were significantly connected to increased waist circumference and insulin resistance.

Could it be that environmental toxins like phthalates are to blame for the increase in overweight, impotent, and pre-diabetic men? The evidence is building, but rather than wait for an official stamp of yes-we-know-enough-now approval, the safest strategy would be to lessen your exposure to these toxins whenever possible.

What You Can Do

- **Skip synthetic fragrances.** Unfortunately, it's not as simple as grabbing "unscented" or "fragrance-free" products, since these phrases often mean that some type of neutral fragrance has been added to buffer the product's actual scent. Look for items scented only with essential oils, like eucalyptus, pine, sage, sandalwood, orange, and coriander. These are all natural, earthy scents that are masculine and strong. Here are a few brands that offer phthalate-free products: Burt's Bees, Dr. Bronner's, Jason Natural Organics, Weleda, Dr. Hauschka, and Aubrey Organics.
- **Outfit your home in nonplastic goods.** Buy shower curtains that are fabric or nylon instead of vinyl. If vinyl is your only option, skip the PVC and reach for those made from ethylene vinyl acetate (EVA) or polyethylene vinyl acetate (PEVA). Dump the plastic spoons, ice cream scoopers, and plastic spatulas and opt for wood, stainless steel, or silicone.

> ### HOT TIP
> Bring an empty stainless-steel or BPA-free bottle with you when you take a flight. Once you're through security, ask a waiter at a bar or coffee shop to fill it with water.

- **Buy package-free foods.** Once you start paying attention to the plastics used today, you will be blown away by how much of what you put into your body has been steeping in plastic for who knows how long. Focus on doing what you can do to avoid plastics, not what you can't do. Purchase "bagged" or fresh produce from the farmers' market or pull from the open stock at the grocery store; carrots, celery, and leafy greens can all be purchased without packaging. Buy foods in bulk, and then store them in glass containers in the refrigerator or, in the case of tomatoes, garlic, and onions, on the kitchen counter.
- **Wood is good.** Pick up wooden cutting boards, bowls, utensils, and toys for kids. Finish items made from untreated wood with mineral, tung, or orange oil to maintain the moisture and create a smooth surface. Wash thoroughly by hand: dishwashers warp wooden bowls and knife handles.

PERSISTENT ORGANIC POLLUTANTS

A blanket term, persistent organic pollutant (POP) describes a long list of synthetic chemicals and pesticides, including dioxins, polychlorinated biphenyls (PCBs), and organotins. What all these substances have in common is that they are persistent, meaning they resist biodegradation—POPs are the cockroaches of the chemical world.

> **MAN MEMO**
>
> Organotins are tin-based chemicals used in pesticides, PVC, silicone, and polyurethane. They leach from the soil into our water supplies and food, disrupting hormonal functions across the food chain, from mollusks to humans.

The POPs maintain their sturdy existence through a process called biomagnification, which means that the concentration of a POP strengthens as it is passed up the food chain—they can grow by 70,000-fold. Once they are absorbed into air, water, or soil, they're easily transported to humans by way of plant and animal consumption. POPs are not water soluble, but they are easily absorbed into fats. For this reason, people who eat large amounts of fatty meat products are more likely to have high levels of these pollutants in their bodies.

Probably the most well known POP is DDT, which has been banned worldwide for nearly thirty years, but is found lingering in millions of human and animal bodies. In men, these persistent pollutants have been shown to strike at the very core. One study of research in this field put it bluntly: "The male reproductive system is vulnerable to the effects of chemicals and physical factors." High exposure to POPs has been linked to decreased sperm quality, lessened libido, lower testosterone levels, and reduced sperm count.

Of all the POPs still in use today, the one scientists are building a big case against is atrazine. This is one of the most commonly used herbicides in the United States, with over 75 million pounds applied annually to crops including corn and soybeans. Atrazine seeps into the ground and by way of agricultural soils and runoff seeps into our water supply. It's so prevalent in our water that it's likely you're taking a sip of it right now. But there are a number of reasons you shouldn't be drinking it. In fact, if I were a gambling man, I'd bet on its becoming the next DDT.

Atrazine exposure has been linked to birth defects and low birth weights, and it has already been banned in Europe. It is also increasingly being linked to reproductive abnormalities in some animal species. Studies involving amphibians, reptiles, mammals, and fish have all revealed the freakish effects of atrazine; these effects include the "feminization" of males—that is, male frogs growing ovaries and male fish demonstrating abnormal gonadal development. In human males, increased exposure to atrazine has been connected to decreased semen quality.

> **MAN MEMO**
>
> A gonad is an organ that produces reproductive cells: the testes in men, the ovaries in women.

Beyond these health effects from atrazine, there's also an alarming link between the ever-growing rates of obesity and general use of atrazine (see "Toxic Obesity" sidebar for more information). In animal tests, chronic exposure to atrazine caused a slower metabolism, increased amounts of visceral fat, and insulin resistance—all without any changes in diet or rate of exercise. In time, it seems, the pieces of the puzzle will come together and reveal atrazine to be a definitive contributor to many of the poor health conditions we're afflicted with today.

> **TOXIC OBESITY**
>
> People have not always been exposed to this many chemicals on a daily basis. Yes, there once was abundant use of unhealthy products like asbestos, lead-based paints, and DDT—all now outlawed—but decades ago the toxic assault wasn't nearly as pervasive.
>
> As scientists and researchers have built an understanding of how dramatic the increase has been, they've also identified parallels between the increased exposure to chemicals and the rise in obesity rates. They've even begun to wonder if exposure to toxins, chemical additives, and POPs is responsible, in large part, for

our obesity epidemic. It's unlikely that a dramatic, sweeping claim assigning *all* the blame to toxins will ever be issued, but some evidence establishes a solid link to major biological disturbances.

For men, I see no reason to wait for that day of judgment to arrive; the evidence of reproductive and sexual abnormalities alone should motivate you to eliminate or minimize your exposure to atrazine and other POPs.

What You Can Do

- **Filter your water.** If you do only one thing, do this. The Natural Resources Defense Council (NRDC) suggests that most household filters that fit onto a tap will scrub your water clean; most important, they will remove atrazine. Visit http://www.nsf.org to find the safest, most effective filters to suit your needs.
- **Cut back on consumption of most animal fats.** Since POPs are fat soluble, the fattier the protein, the greater the likelihood of exposure to atrazine. Since fish and fish oil in particular have so many other benefits, for your animal protein needs, purchase wild-caught fish over farmed. Farmed fish have been shown to have higher levels of POPs.
- **Wash your hands.** The same habits that help curb your exposure to germs also help wash away evidence of toxic exposure. Wash your hands thoroughly and often—use soap and running water for at least 20 seconds. Skip the antibacterial soaps, however. Many of them contain triclosan, which has been shown to have endocrine-disrupting effects in animals.
- **Drop your shoes at the door.** Many of the pollutants we carry into our homes travel in by way of the soles of our shoes. Removing your shoes by the front door will cut down on the number of polluted particles you bring home. Plus, leaving your shoes outside will help keep things a bit cleaner in the home, which no one will complain about.
- **Stay up to date on the dirty dozen.** The Environmental Working Group (EWG) releases two lists each year, one indicating which fruits and vegetables should be purchased as organic, the other suggesting which ones can be bought conventionally. Most important to follow is their "Dirty Dozen"—the twelve fruits and vegetables ranked highest in pesticide content (see full list on page 157). You can also visit the EWG's site for updated versions of the list: http://www.ewg.org/foodnews/summary/.

DON'T FORGET THE MEDICINE CABINET

As you take an inventory of your environment—and a good solid look at your daily exposure to plastics and pollutants—it's important not to overlook another possible threat to your waistline: what's in your medicine cabinet. Whether you are depressed (and taking Elavil, Tofranil, or Paxil), anxious (Clozaril, Risperadal), diabetic (Avandia, Actose, Diabeta), or hypertensive (Hytrin, Inderal), you may be setting yourself up for weight gain. Researchers have revealed that patients can gain up to 22 pounds a year as a result of a prescription medication. Here are many of the common medications associated with weight gain:

Antidepressants

Lithium (Eskalith, Lithobid, etc.)
Valproic acid (Depakote, etc.)
Isocarboxazid (Marplan)
Phenelzine (Nardil)
Tranylcypromine (Parnate)
Mirtazapine (Remeron)
Citalopram (Celexa)
Fluoxetine (Prozac)
Paroxetine (Paxil)

Sertraline (Zoloft)
Amitriptyline (Elavil)
Clomipramine (Anafranil)
Desipramine (Norpramin)
Doxepin (Sinequan)
Imipramine (Tofranil)
Maprotiline (Ludiomil)
Nortriptyline (Pamelor)

Antihistamines

Cetirizine (Zyrtec)
Diphenhydramine (Benadryl)

Fexofenadine (Allegra)
Hydroxyzine (Vistaril, etc.)

Antihypertensives

Prazosin (Minipress)
Terazosin (Hytrin)
Atenolol (Tenormin)
Propranolol (Inderal)
Clonidine (Catapres)

Guanabenz (Wytensin)
Guanethidine (Ismelin)
Methyldopa (Aldomet, etc.)
Minoxidil (Loniten)

Antipsychotics

Chlorpromazine (Thorazine)
Fluphenazine (Prolixin, etc.)

Haloperidol (Haldol)
Perphenazine (Trilafon)

Thioridazine (Mellaril)
Thiothixene (Navane)
Trifluoperazine (Stelazine)
Aripiprazole (Abilify)
Clozapine (Clozaril)

Olanzapine (Zyprexa)
Quetiapine (Seroquel)
Risperidone (Risperdal)
Ziprasidone (Geodon)

Hormones

Corticosteroids
Megestrol (Megace)
Insulin

Hypoglycemics

Nateglinide (Starlix)
Repaglinide (Prandin)
Chlorpropamide (Diabinese)
Glimepiride (Amaryl)
Glipizide (Glucotrol)

Glyburide (Glynase, etc.)
Tolbutamide (Orinase)
Pioglitazone (Actos)
Rosiglitazone (Avandia)

Anticonvulsants/Mood Stabilizers

Carbamazepine (Tegretol, etc.)
Gabapentin (Neurontin)
Pregabalin (Lyrica)

In addition, some medications are coated in toxic phthalates. These prescription and over-the-counter medications are known to contain phthalates:

- Brompheniramine
- Carbamazepine
- Diltiazem
- Erythromycin
- Ketoprofen
- Mesalamine

- Omeprazole
- Potassium chloride
- Propranolol
- Ranitidine
- Verapamil

Other medications may be covered in phthalates, too. If you are currently taking medication, especially one for long-term use, ask your pharmacist if it contains phthalates; if so, request a phthalate-free alternative. When buying over-the-counter (OTC) medications, ask about terms like "delayed release," "controlled release," "time release," "targeted release," and "enteric coatings." Pills with these phrases on their labels are more likely to be sealed in endocrine-disrupting coating.

If you're taking one or more of the above medications, it's likely it was prescribed or suggested for a good medical reason. So, I'm not telling you to stop taking it; I'm recommending that you ask questions about it and develop an informed opinion.

The good news is that you may not always be a slave to those pill bottles. Fitness and weight loss, especially belly-fat loss, can liberate you from the need to take medications for chronic conditions like high cholesterol, diabetes, and high blood pressure. Regular exercise is especially effective at reducing medication dependency (more on exercise in Chapter 3).

It does not have to be your fate to be dependent on medication. Dietary changes alone can alter gene expression, and amazingly, you can control how your genes work by changing what you eat. Your health is fluid and responsive, not concrete, so don't make assumptions and always be ready to ask questions, both in your own research and of your doctor (#mylifemyhealth).

WHEN YOUR BEST IS GOOD ENOUGH

I'll be the first to admit that discussing toxins and environmental pollutants is like opening Pandora's box. This is why, at the end of the day, my advice is anchored to one important point: do not let perfection be the enemy of good (hat tip: Voltaire).

THE TWO SIMPLEST STEPS TO REDUCING TOXIC EXPOSURE:

- Wash your hands regularly with good, old-fashioned, unscented bar soap and running water for 20 seconds plus.
- Drink filtered water.

Take action now by implementing the easiest steps of those I've shared with you and you will soon help boost your reproductive and sexual health, as well as minimize your propensity for dangerous weight gain. Many of these tips are especially important if you are actively trying to have kids—the fewer toxins you swim in, the stronger your little swimmers will be.

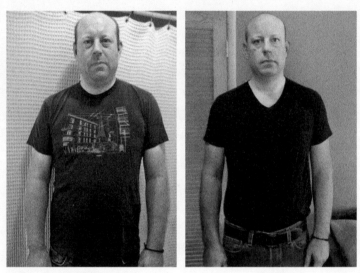

Day I   Day 24

REFUEL SUCCESS
Name: **Jason T.**
Age: **37**
Weight Loss in 24 Days: **I6 pounds**
Waist Loss: **5 inches**

Jason T. had wanted to lose weight for a long time, but felt stuck in a rut. Then, something happened that made him realize he had to change. "I was taking a picture in a Polo shirt for my company website, and when I looked at the pictures, I had extra skin around my neck and lots of belly fat," he recalls. "Worse, my chest was pointy, like I had boobs. I had to tape down the points so I could take the picture. At that point I knew I needed to lose weight."

His weight gain was gradual. "I think I unconsciously avoided seeing my appearance. I never really looked in mirrors; just when I was washing my hands or getting ready quickly, but I never really got the whole picture." Jason found himself spending more time at happy hours, socializing and drinking a lot, which led to eating a lot, too. "It became more of a crutch, I think; there's a sort of gratification in eating and drinking whatever you want."

He had tried a lot of different ways to drop weight: cleanses, all vegetables, raw foods, no carbs, lots of exercise. "I've always put on weight easily and never been a big exerciser." He was looking for something he could stick with long term when Refuel came along.

What Changed

"I had a lot going on when I first started the plan," he says. "I was busy with work; I had seminars to attend and company in town for business."

Still, when he stepped onto the scale on day 6, he realized he had lost 4 pounds. "It really came by surprise—I didn't prepare well and still it was very easy."

The fast results were motivating, kicking him into full gear with the program. "I made sure I was drinking as much citrus water as I could, refilling with filtered water and carrying a stainless-steel bottle. I tried to stay away from plastics, especially when it involved heating or hot things. I ate in-shell pistachios for snacks, which prevent eating by the handful, and a variety of fish, and skipped sauces on meats."

He didn't stop going out or eating at restaurants, but he made changes to how he ordered. "I just tried to make the smartest choice—chicken with lemon and capers and extra vegetables, no potatoes or starches."

Since Jason has diverticulitis, he still needed to make sure he was getting enough fiber despite keeping an eye on carbs. "I ate tons of vegetables and salads, and my water intake was huge—I never used to drink enough water."

What's Better Now

"It got me out of my rut," says Jason. "I realized it's somewhat depressing—to not be where you want to be mentally and physically."

The changes were noticeable in just ten days. "I was working a lot and didn't see my friends during that time. When they saw me, I heard 'Wow!' They were shocked at how much weight I had lost already."

Everything seems to be changing, in a good way. "My face and body look thinner and healthier, my pants are practically falling off—it's definitely motivating. And it's nice that people are noticing."

A big benefit for Jason was improved sleep. "I rarely used to wake up feeling well rested," he says. "I have sleep apnea and bouts of acid reflux, but I've noticed I'm sleeping much better and I'm not experiencing the scary moment where I wake up choking from reflux."

Best Tips
- **Establish return-to foods.** "I made a lot of great salads: lettuce with some type of meat, avocado, tomato, and crumbled feta with a squeeze of Meyer lemon on top—I would also use these in my water. Or, I'd pick up broccoli slaw and grab pistachios and almonds for snacks."
- **Try something new.** "I started adding hemp seeds to my salads and to Greek yogurt—they're really good-tasting and they add omega-3s."
- **Don't skip meals.** "I made sure to eat three meals a day—yogurt, sometimes with fruit, or eggs for breakfast, a bread-free lunch, and a big salad for dinner. And I was never really hungry."

3

THE .350 AVERAGE

How Better Sleep, Strategic Exercise,
and Stress Optimization Can Create All-Star Health

If your waist circumference extends beyond 40 inches, you've done some work to create that belly—it hasn't just popped up (or out) overnight. I could list the questions that help me diagnose your specific path to weight gain, but the contributing factors are likely the same for most guys. Besides paying attention to diet and toxic exposure, there are three other areas you cannot ignore if you want to lose the gut and rebuild your testosterone: sleep, exercise, and stress optimization.

These three areas of your life are so pivotal that I've incorporated distinct strategies for mastering each one. And since you can't have mastery without practice, I teach you how to get there. Like heading to the driving range to work on your golf swing, you can work on getting better rest, learn how to exercise smarter, and improve your response to stress.

I've created the Rest, Exercise, and Unwind protocol (RE-UP) to put you on the right track; you'll see the RE-UP steps for each phase of the program. But first, let's have a look at why these three areas of body improvement are essential for burning calories while you sleep—literally.

REST FOR THE WEARY

The notion of getting "a good night's sleep" seems a bit quaint or nostalgic—it's what we were told when we were growing up: to get sleep before a big game, a major test, or a long road trip. At that time, it was practically insulting to be told to get some sleep. Now, if you're like most guys, you only wish someone would make the time for you to get to bed early.

> ## MAN MEMO
> A full 63 percent of Americans feel that their sleep needs aren't being met. Buck the zombie trend: get at least seven hours of sleep a night. (#notazombie)

Sleep remains, as ever, a critical period for rejuvenation, rebuilding, and metabolic balancing. Today, it's also a much-needed balm against the chronic electronic assault on the eyes. (Think about it—how often are you *not* looking at some type of screen?) We often dismiss going to bed late or getting too little sleep as harmless, something to be managed with more coffee. But chronic lack of sleep is a culprit responsible for more than the current boon for caffeine providers. Many in the medical community believe that chronic sleep deprivation is a significant contributor to the obesity epidemic.

Over the last fifty years, people's average daily sleep duration has been truncated by about two hours. This change is significant, since the risks for disease and weight gain jump up a great deal when you compare, say, seven hours of sleep to five hours.

What exactly happens that is so important when you sleep? Well, a better question would be, What *doesn't* happen? The amount of sleep you get plays a role in appetite function, immune health, growth-hormone and testosterone synthesis, tissue development and repair, memory storage and other critical brain functions, and cardiovascular health.

> **MAN MEMO**
> Since you make testosterone while you sleep, your T levels are highest in the morning. Having a blood test to get your T levels checked? Schedule it for before 8:00 A.M.

When you sleep, you make growth hormone, which is needed for maintaining normal metabolism, energy levels, and libido—and for building muscle. Less sleep means less muscle, more hunger, and more weight gain. Participants in a sleep study who slept between five and six hours a night were likely to consume nearly 550 calories more than they did when they got eight hours of sleep. Considering that it takes only an extra 50 to 100 calories a day to lead to gradual weight gain, you can imagine what more than 500 calories will do—it's being put on the fast track to fat.

> **FIVE UNCONVENTIONAL (IF IMPRACTICAL) WAYS TO BURN 550 CALORIES**
>
> • Play the accordion for three and a half hours.
> • Chop wood for a little over an hour.
> • Shave for four hours.
> • Milk a cow by hand for two hours.
> • Play miniature golf for two hours.

Less sleep, a monster appetite, and more weight gain often occur one after the other. Without adequate rest, your body's pathways of communication break down, and you continue to eat though you're full and your hunger seems to never be satisfied. You stay hungry even when you eat a Snickers bar or a whole bag of chips or most of the leftover macaroni salad (why is there macaroni in a salad, anyway?).

Even bigger trouble is hiding in the link between diminished quality and quantity of sleep, on the one hand, and glucose tolerance and insulin sensitivity, on the other. Prolonged sleep loss can throw a monkey wrench into these critical fueling functions.

With compromised glucose tolerance and impaired insulin sensitivity comes the risk of pre-diabetes and then the full-blown manifestation of the disease. Because pre-diabetes and diabetes (just points on a continuum of insulin resistance) are such common conditions today, people tend to not see them as the red flags they are. Diabetes can cause nerve damage, blindness, severe fatigue, gangrene and resulting amputations, erectile dysfunction, and kidney damage, among other serious health problems—it is not to be treated lightly.

> ### MAN MEMO
> Doctors don't always test for diabetes. If you feel extra thirsty or often need to urinate, or you want to eat all the time for no reason, be proactive and schedule a fasting blood-glucose test or a glycohemoglobin test with your doctor or pharmacist, or do one yourself with a drugstore glucometer (or a smartphone app). You'll find recommended models and kits at www.drjohnlapuma.com.

A common misconception about sleep is that, somehow, the body magically adjusts to dealing with sleep deprivation. It doesn't. What really happens is that the sleep-deprived person becomes oblivious to the ways that sleep affects daily performance or productivity. That blunder you made in the PowerPoint presentation at work or the sore thumb you got from hitting it instead of a 16-penny nail could be a result of diminished function from lack of sleep, especially invaluable REM sleep.

> ### MAN MEMO
> Your major voluntary muscle groups are paralyzed during REM sleep, which is why being awoken from a deep sleep can be disorienting—you literally can't move your arms or legs for a few seconds.

University of Pennsylvania School of Medicine researchers found that sleeping between four and six hours per night for fourteen consecutive days creates the same drops in cognitive performance as experiencing total sleep deprivation for one or two days.

If you think back to college, or work all-nighters (I hope you're not pulling them now), you can recall the dazed sort of delirium that sets in. You're putting yourself in that same state when you consistently sleep five hours or less at night. The trick is that your body might not give obvious signs of sleepiness, even though your alertness and memory are being compromised. This means that someone or something else, like your boss or the lightpost on the side of the road, is going to notice your fatigue before you do.

In men, prolonged sleep loss has been linked to lower testosterone levels, with one study finding a 10 to 15 percent testosterone drop in men who slept only five hours a night. Sleep deprivation in men has also been shown to increase levels of an angry, inflammatory protein called tumor necrosis factor (TNF). As with estrogen, men need a little TNF to perform important functions, but too much is associated with chronic inflammatory disorders, such as rheumatoid arthritis. And chronically elevated levels of TNF have been linked to insulin resistance, high blood pressure, and heart disease.

For most men, the ideal amount of sleep is more than seven hours but less than nine hours. That's hours spent sleeping, not just hours spent in bed. If you go to bed early enough but spend half the night with your eyes glued to the TV or the ceiling, that time doesn't count.

> **MAN MEMO**
> A neck circumference greater than 17 inches often signals a sleep apnea sufferer. In studies, larger neck circumference has also been shown to have a strong link to abdominal obesity. Here's a hint: if you tie a standard necktie so that the front and back are even once tied, and the tie then rises above your belly button, measure your neck—and get checked for sleep apnea.

If you've done battle with sleep apnea or insomnia, getting seven hours of sleep might seem only the stuff of dreams; you might be inclined to think the solution is sleep medication. Well, even though I'm not your doctor, I am a doctor; and I've seen some scary stuff out there about sleeping pills. One study revealed that sleeping-pill poppers were more than four times likely to die over a two-and-a-half-year period than people not taking pills; taking even just eighteen pills over the course of a year was linked to a greater risk of death. Researchers similarly found that those taking sleeping aids were 35 percent more likely to develop lung, lymphatic, prostate, or colon cancer. There is a better way.

> ## ▶ MAN MEMO
> Sleeping pills are usually only modestly effective. If taken regularly for several months, they up a person's sleep times by an average of only 30 minutes.

The Sleep Thieves

Approximately 12 million people in the United States have some form of sleep apnea, and as a man, you are twice or three times as likely to have it. At least one in twenty-five men has this breathing disorder, according to a 1994 study, and one recent estimate put the prevalence closer to one in four. People over age 65 are the most vulnerable.

At least four of five men with sleep apnea don't know they have it; and for many, it's a vicious circle. Their obesity puts them at risk, and their sleep apnea lowers their testosterone levels. Peak testosterone levels occur just before REM sleep, which means that interrupted or unconsolidated sleep can slow or even put the brakes on T production.

You have obstructive sleep apnea—the most common type—if your breathing is obstructed for at least 10 seconds at a time while you're sleeping. The three cardinal signs all begin with *s*: snoring, sleepiness, and your significant other telling you that you stopped breathing while you slept.

If you're a loud snorer, you should get tested. Symptoms of sleep apnea include choking during sleep, feeling chronically unrested, restless sleep, and daytime sleepiness. Of course, the clearest sign of all might be getting a shove in the middle of the night, accompanied by the command "Stop snoring!"

Other common causes of insomnia are restless leg syndrome, nocturnal leg cramps, frequent urination, and heartburn. Here are a few quick tips for treating several of these causes:

- **For leg cramps:** Take hot baths, get massages, and be sure to move around enough during the day. Try wrapping a towel around your toes with your cramped leg extended and gently pulling the towel toward you to ease muscle tightness. Also, be sure you are drinking enough water throughout the day, as dehydration alone can cause muscle cramping.

- **Nighttime nature calls:** Limit consumption of beverages two hours before bedtime (see advice about caffeine-containing beverages, page 54) and be sure to get your blood glucose and prostate checked—diabetes and prostate enlargement are sometimes signaled by frequent urination.
- **Your heart's on fire:** You could have gastroesophageal reflux disease (GERD), which inflames the lining of the esophagus and can cause coughing, choking, or indigestion. Weight loss will ease these symptoms, and so too will not eating or drinking alcohol three hours prior to bedtime.

Sleep apnea is under-diagnosed in medical practice and is both serious and treatable. Continuous positive airway pressure (CPAP) is often used with some success when sleep apnea is tested for and treated, and patients feel better.

But the good news is that if you've been diagnosed with sleep apnea or have insomnia, or both, Refuel will help you drop them like bad habits. In fact, several men who have Refueled reported reduced snoring (or reduced complaints of sawing logs). Since over half of sleep apnea cases are caused or worsened by excess weight, dropping fat from all over your body will certainly help you get uninterrupted sleep. And if you can eat to beat sleep apnea, would you rather do that than wear an oxygen mask?

If not sleeping pills, then maybe a few cocktails before bed or an intense workout will help, right? Nope. Alcohol consumption late at night just leads to tossing and turning, and an overall diminished quality of sleep. And evening workouts can overstimulate the body and make it tough to come down from the endorphins and adrenaline.

Getting enough good-quality sleep will take more than willpower. Solving a sleep problem takes a strategic approach, which you'll find in the RE-UP sections in each phase of the Refuel™ program; see Part Three. Generally speaking, here's what's critical to getting great shut-eye:

- **A dark room.** Sleep experts suggest treating your sleeping space like a cave. Keep it dark, quiet, and cool, and use your bed only for sleep and sex.

- **Limited electronic exposure.** Shut down and power off all electronic gadgets and TVs at least five minutes prior to bed; ideally, you should build up to an hour of screen-free time prior to bed.
- **A relatively cool room.** Aim to create a sleeping temperature between 65 and 72 degrees. If you're cold, pull on some socks, as your cold feet will sometimes wake you up in the middle of the night.
- **A slightly raised pillow.** If you suffer from sleep apnea or GERD, raising your pillow just a few inches can help keep the airways clear and prevent sleep disturbances.
- **No caffeine after 2:00 P.M.** Caffeine has an elimination half-life of between 1.5 and 9.5 hours; a person's sensitivity varies. The half-life is exactly what it sounds like: how long it takes to flush half of the substance out of your system. If you drink caffeine and experience sleep disturbances, try setting an afternoon cutoff time for yourself.

Insomnia is a killer. Exercise is a cure. Studies have found that, across the board, exercise improves sleep. Whether you're young, old, or middle-aged, whether you lift weights or have a regular cardio habit, exercise will inspire better rest. Exercise has been shown to not only increase sleep times but also improve "sleep efficiency"—this means that you're more likely to hit the pillow and drift right off, rather than waste precious sleep time tossing and turning.

> ▶ **HOT TIP**
> Finish any intense workout at least four hours before bedtime. This will give your body time to cool down completely and prepare itself for sleep.

This brings us to the next part of the Rest, Exercise, and Unwind protocol—exercise. If the word *exercise* triggers a reflexive list of "don't dos" and "can't dos," I've got a counterattack that's guaranteed to beat down those excuses.

EXERCISE

Hippocrates once wrote, "Eating alone will not keep a man well; he must also take exercise. For food and exercise, while possessing opposite qualities, yet work together to produce health."

This is what I like to think of as evergreen advice: despite the fact that it was written thousands of years ago, it remains profoundly true today. Can you drop fat by only changing what you eat? Yes, but you won't look and feel as good as you deserve. Nor will you get the other benefits: better cardiovascular health, stronger and bigger muscles, better sleep, better sex, improved mood, higher testosterone levels, enhanced mitochondrial function, and sustained weight loss.

STAND UP FOR YOUR HEALTH

Sitting for extended periods of time isn't great for the body. You don't have to read the research to know that's true; you've probably discovered that when you sit for a long time, your body becomes stiff, achy, and filled with all sorts of twinges and knots. Internally, you get all tied up, too.

Here's a quick summary of the research: the more you sit, the sooner you die, irrespective of whether you work out.

Before I dive into why you need to get physical, I want to step back a minute and reiterate an important point about exercise. *Exercise alone will not create a profound loss of pounds.* From a pure energy-exchange perspective, you can re-consume all the calories you've burned in an entire day of exercise by eating just half of a Marie Callender's chicken potpie or a big serving of chili cheese fries.

In fact, you can outeat any amount of exercise—which is why it's essential for you to have your mental game in place. I want you to think of exercise as your point guard and the food elements of this plan as your power forward. You need exercise for the movement—the action, because it can drive the game—but ultimately the exercise gets more assists than points. Your diet, on the other hand, gets in the paint and really mixes things up. It becomes a steady scorer and makes you an all-star.

There's another reason I want you to approach exercise with a realistic sense of precisely what it will do for your body; that way, you'll avoid the disappointment of unmet expectations. The problem is that exercise expectations are a bit warped in the fitness industry's marketing to men: "Six-pack abs in 10 minutes!" "Add two inches to your biceps in just seconds a day!" You get the idea.

> ## MOVE NOW
>
> Even if you're an otherwise active person, sitting for long periods of time can increase waist circumference, raise inflammatory proteins, affect glucose and insulin functions, and lead to increased triglycerides. Prevent these occurrences by standing up or walking around at least once an hour, even if it's just for I minute. Get up, stretch, and rest your eyes by staring out into empty space for a moment. Take phone calls while standing (make the phone ring your trigger to stand up).

In reality, building muscle takes time, but strength improvements can come quickly. Women have an advantage over men when it comes to exercise and fat loss: their bodies are somehow programmed to burn fat first when exercising; men's bodies are not.

Where you do have the advantage is in how *much* fat you lose while exercising. Men have been shown to lose more fat than women when they've created the same energy deficit while exercising (number of calories consumed vs. number of calories expended).

You also have an ability to create "preferential" fat loss with exercise. That is, *Medicine & Science in Sports & Exercise* reported on a study showing that thirty overweight men who completed four months of training dropped a significant amount of abdominal fat, while maintaining and improving their muscle mass.

> ## MAN MEMO
>
> Myth or fact? A pound of muscle weighs more than a pound of fat. Myth. A pound is a pound. The difference between them is in volume: I pound of muscle is like a tightly wound baseball; I pound of fat is about the size of a child's squishy soccer ball.

Additional research conducted by French physicians revealed that exercising as little as three times per week, with two days of that exercise performed mostly at high intensity, can effectively target visceral fat. After two months of exercise, measurements of study participants revealed that 48 percent of their weight loss had involved visceral fat—it was as though their bodies were literally programmed by exercise to drop the riskiest kind of fat.

> ## THE HEFTY PRICE OF INACTIVITY
>
> With exercise, the phrase "something is better than nothing" rings true. Researchers working to reveal a connection between exercise and belly fat found that in nonexercising control-group members, the level of visceral fat rose by nearly 10 percent in just six months. This is why I like to apply the 5-minute rule to exercise: complete something for 5 minutes and then if you want to stop, you can. It's a manipulative mind game, but it works: once you develop a rhythm, your endorphins kick in and the exercise begins to feel good. Try it—I dare you not to stop.

Another main advantage of exercise is that once you exercise, your body will continue to burn fat for a very long time during recovery: this is known as the *afterburn*. Despite losing out to women in the initial-fat-loss arena, men's bodies have an incredible ability to keep burning fat for up to 21 hours *after* an exercise session. Fat burning continues even though you're eating meals and sleeping. I can't think of a patient I've met who doesn't want to burn fat while eating dinner or sitting on the couch.

When you exercise regularly, you will not only promote fat loss but you'll also improve just about every other part of your health. Habitual exercise has been shown to:

- Boost immune health by increasing white blood cell count
- Help the body rid itself of toxins and carcinogens
- Improve the ability to manage stress and respond to anger
- Speed up healing
- Create more resilient, age-resistant brain cells
- Increase levels of growth hormone
- Promote cleansing and "housekeeping" of cells, which helps your body fight disease
- Improve mood and overall outlook on life

These are all convincing reasons to start walking, lifting, or cycling, but they don't stamp out the most often cited excuse for not exercising: lack of time.

I know that almost every man reading this feels he's constantly battling time; too many competing demands and opposing directions can cut out the small section of a day that you've reserved for just you. That's why we're going to use the most efficient exercise method available to ensure that you can make this important commitment to yourself: burst training. This is also referred to as interval training, sprint training, or high-intensity interval training (HIIT).

These methods vary slightly from one another, but they are all based on the same idea: quick bursts of going nearly all-out, followed by longer intervals of mild pace or rest. Competitive athletes have been using interval training for hundreds of years; it helps create quick, dramatic improvements in cardiovascular strength and endurance, and it teaches the body to work more efficiently.

The benefits can be experienced by beginning exercisers, too. The key is to find what's considered your maximum effort and your mild to moderate effort. With burst training, you accelerate progress in your biological and metabolic functions; you teach your body to take in and utilize oxygen like a champ, which in turn fires up your caloric burn.

Burst training has been shown in studies to increase the secretion of growth hormone, with greater increases as the intensity of exercise performance goes up. This is especially beneficial if part of your goal in the Refuel program is to drop belly fat—abdominal fat is known to reduce circulating levels of natural growth hormone. Skip synthetic growth hormone, which comes with the risk of side effects, and try first this smarter way of training. If done correctly, burst training will also help you:

1. Burn more calories in less time
2. Reduce occurrence of overuse injuries
3. Avoid boredom and burnout
4. Build lean, fat-burning muscle faster

Studies have shown that benefits, such as increased cardio performance and improved insulin sensitivity, can be experienced in as little as two weeks, or about six sessions of burst training. Interval training has also been rated in research as more "enjoyable" than moderate exercise. The more a person enjoys something, the more likely he is to do it. That means you.

> **HOT TIP**
>
> Treadmills lead to more trips to the ER than any other exercise equipment. To prevent injury (to your ego, too), stay focused: keep your eyes off that woman in tight shorts, stop texting, and if your iPod falls, let it. Once it lands, stop the treadmill and go pick it up. Replacing a broken iPod or cell phone is significantly cheaper than a hospital visit. (#deadlytmill)

When you get to the phases part of the program in Part Three, you'll have detailed instructions on how to perform your burst training sessions. I've included both cardiovascular and resistance components, which work together to encourage complete health through strength building, fat loss, and optimal heart function.

I should say *almost* complete health, since we have one more part of the RE-UP to get to: the supremely important skill of knowing how to unwind. While you won't ever be able to erase stress entirely, you can learn how to better respond to it, which will minimize the toll it takes on your health, your work, and your family, and you will become more productive in your daily life. I'll show you how it's done.

THE GREAT UNWIND: HOW TO MASTER YOUR MINDSET AND CONTROL CHRONIC STRESS

While you're less likely than your female counterparts to report problems in managing chronic stress, you are just as susceptible, if not more so, to its health consequences. Most men are aware that the buildup of daily pressures can have a significant effect on their health; 78 percent of men surveyed in a poll done by the American Psychological Association agreed that stress had a "very strong/strong" impact on their health.

Despite acknowledging this, men are less likely to make a direct connection between long-term stress and medical issues and/or unhealthy behaviors or habits. But more men, when compared with women, have muscle tightness and hypertension. They're also more likely to display aggressive behavior and to abuse drugs and alcohol. These problems impact job performance, home life, and family. And they are created or exacerbated by chronic stress.

There's huge pressure on men to put up a strong front and to endure the takedowns, the financial worries, the long hours, the tasks that need to be accomplished just to get through the day. The question isn't whether you can handle everything life tosses at you; it's whether you can handle it without its dramatically deteriorating your health or causing a significant reduction in your quality of life, your work performance, and your relationships.

When you experience chronic stress, you produce high levels of the stress hormone cortisol. Cortisol has its purposes, one of which is to surge in the morning to make sure you're alert and awake when you need to be. Under normal circumstances, it then dips back down in the evening and reaches its lowest point a few hours into your nightly sleep.

But when cortisol levels don't recede in the evening, during sleep, or—worse—ever, your body will signal you to reach for high-fat or high-sugar foods and will deposit fat deep in your abdominal region. Long term, persistently high cortisol levels can also cause a weakened immune system by combating your ability to create short-term inflammation.

> ### MAN MEMO
> You need some acute inflammation: in certain cases, it's a good thing. When redness and swelling occur as a response to injury, your body is trying to minimize the damage and begin the healing process.

Severe stress can manifest in a number of measurable, physical ways: weight gain in the abdominal region, chest pains, high blood pressure, elevated heart rate, muscle aches, lack of libido, erectile dysfunction, digestive issues, heartburn, and insomnia. It can mean reduced ability to concentrate, an iffy memory, and a constant feeling of shortness of breath.

There are more ways the wrong mindset can hold you back or change and alter your daily experience of life. If you feel perpetually unmotivated, irritated, fatigued, or unable to sleep (different sides of the same coin), or you feel the need to drown your sorrows regularly—that is, you drink yourself to sleep—you are most likely experiencing symptoms of chronic stress. The problem is that it could be killing you, not softly but slowly, and sabotaging your work, your family, and your health.

> **HOT TIP**
> Have a short fuse? Grab a stick of gum before you blow it. Gum chewing has been shown to help relieve anxiety and reduce stress.

With the RE-UP, you will learn how to improve these parameters from several different angles, and you will see the specific instructions for mastering chronic stress within each phase. And learning how to improve productivity, increase equilibrium, and retool your mindset to master chronic stress will help improve your relationships. That brings its own benefits: strong social connections have been linked to improved quality of life and greater longevity. You'll be more efficient and effective at work and at home. A better mindset will help you drop belly fat, lower blood pressure and cholesterol, and boost heart health. That's a win all around.

For now, I want to explain why these methods are so effective at minimizing the wear and tear of a tough day.

Breathing Techniques

Well-known health and wellness expert Dr. Andrew Weil once said, "If I had to limit my advice on healthier living to just one tip, it would be simply to learn how to breathe correctly." These are wise words. When we're stressed, breathing often happens in quick, short spurts. This leads to tight muscles, clouded thinking, irritability, and feelings of anxiety and panic. No one makes smart choices from this state.

When you feel tightness build in your chest or have an overwhelming sense of angst, pause and try taking a *4-7-8 Belly Breath*: inhale for 4 counts through your nose, hold for 7 counts, exhale through your mouth for 8 counts. Repeat four times. You'll notice an immediate release of pressure. From here, aim to operate from that little patch of calm you just created in your brain. Repeat this easy-to-master breathing exercise throughout the day as often as needed. More on this later.

Protein in the Morning

Say no in the morning to starchy sugar buns and high-carbohydrate, sugary cereals, and make sure you have food with enough protein at breakfast. When you eat foods rich in protein in the morning, you set the stage for a balanced day, at least as it relates to your appetite, energy levels, and hormone functions. Protein takes longer to digest than carbs or fat, so you will feel fuller longer. Plus your brain and tissues will thank you: protein gets broken down into amino acids, which your body uses to rebuild itself. Your co-workers will be grateful, too. Skipping the high-sugar start to a day will help prevent the sudden energy crash at 9:30 A.M.; try Easy Homemade Breakfast Sausage (page 225) instead, and you'll be sharp and alert throughout the morning.

> ## MAN MEMO
> Amino acids are the building blocks of proteins. When you eat foods with protein, your body breaks this protein down into amino acids, which are then used to repair and build muscles and other important tissues. (#buildmuscle)

Hit the Mat

Studies have shown that yoga can reduce a man's blood pressure, lower cholesterol and triglyceride levels, and improve overall quality of life. A Swedish study found that yoga reduced feelings of anger and exhaustion and improved blood pressure measures, lowered heart rate, and decreased levels of inflammation throughout the body.

For yoga, I recommend taking a beginning class at your local gym—gyms often offer classes that are much less intimidating than those you might find at a yoga studio. Most gyms and studios rent mats, so you don't have to make that investment until you know yoga is something you'll continue.

> **HOT TIP**
> Public yoga and workout mats are hotbeds of germs: jock itch, plantar warts, and staph bacteria can all reside there. Most gyms have antibacterial sprays for wiping down exercise equipment after use. It's worth 2 minutes of your time to spray a paper towel and wipe a borrowed mat down before you use it as well.

Have More Sex

I know I'm preaching to the choir, but let me tell you why you should be having more sex: it's one of the best ways to relieve stress and improve your ability to manage stress.

> **HOT TIP**
> Yes, you can show this page to your partner. Actually, you should.

Having intercourse has been linked with lowered blood pressure and better responses to stress. This effect stems from the release of oxytocin during and immediately after sex. Oxytocin is like the body's natural form of Xanax, and it can have a long-lasting sedative effect.

There is a chance that sex has actually been a source of stress in your life. Being overweight or obese has a well-established link to decreased libido, problems with erections, and male infertility. You may be no stranger to these facts.

The great news: even a 10 percent weight loss rapidly and significantly improves erectile function. And often, the more weight loss, generally speaking, the more sex. Having a serious sex drive, and then being able to get it up, make more sex not just possible but a reality.

PUTTING IT ALL TOGETHER

There's a reason the Rest, Exercise, and Unwind protocol includes those three areas of your life. Even though they are three separate skills, they are three integral parts of a whole. Better sleep and more exercise will lead to better mind-body control; better control will create better sleep and more energy. When you implement strategies to create improvements across the board, you will have earned yourself a spot in the big game. Just remember, though: you've got to eat to score.

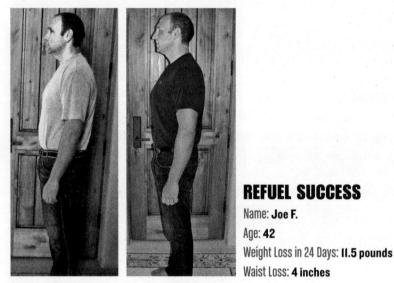

Day I   Day 24

REFUEL SUCCESS
Name: **Joe F.**
Age: **42**
Weight Loss in 24 Days: **11.5 pounds**
Waist Loss: **4 inches**

The Weight Gain

Joe F.'s weight gain, he says, started at birth: "I was blessed with the fat gene; just genetically prone to be heavy." Carrying around extra weight seemed to be another inherited trait, like brown eyes and hair, courtesy of his Italian heritage.

It wasn't a legacy he was happy to carry on. "I would try different things to change, but my weight yo-yoed significantly—between 270 and 185." A deep love of great food and wines, he says, didn't help things much.

Five months before starting Refuel, Joe had decided it was time to drop some pounds. "I adopted a general 'eat better and exercise more' kind of plan. It was working, but I felt myself starting to slip and I had hit a plateau. That's when Refuel came along and really rejuvenated me."

What Changed

Before starting the plan, Joe would sometimes start the day with a bowl of cereal. He'd pour without paying attention, just filling the bowl. "I really had no idea how much I was eating," he says. "I looked at the label, which said ¾ cup was a serving, and measured that much out—it was eye opening how much more I was eating."

He didn't by any means become a fanatical portion monitor: "I just started paying attention more. You realize that you can eat a lot less food and still feel satisfied."

Joe found that keeping an eye on carbs two days a week was a strategy he could stick with. "For two days a week, I feel like I'm really focused on 50 grams, but after that I loosen up a bit—it worked great and it's a strategy that now feels like part of my life."

It helped that meals at home didn't change much: Joe is the father of two teenagers, and they ate mostly according to the plan, too. "It wasn't disruptive to my family—we would have roasted Brussels sprouts instead of mashed potatoes, or a little couscous instead of a lot of rice. It was mostly about carbohydrate substitutions that were easy to make."

Joe credits his wife with helping him stick to the plan and being open to adopting simple swaps. "She used to make me a smoothie in the morning with bananas, yogurt, and orange juice—obviously high in sugar and carbs. Now she'll add ricotta, coconut milk, and berries. We didn't have to cut anything out; we just had to learn how to make it differently."

Another part of his success came from taking the general Refuel guidelines and using them to improve his habits. "I ride dressage and I used to think of that as my exercise for the day, but then I came to the part of the plan that addressed intensity," says Joe. "I could never say after my riding that I had worked out at a level 8 intensity. Asking myself that question helped me make changes—I started running more and with high-intensity intervals."

What's Better Now

"I used to wake up in the middle of the night with heartburn and muscle aches—just an overall heaviness made me sore. Now, I sleep better and I feel and look noticeably better."

His wardrobe has improved, too, especially since his combined weight loss is up to over 60 pounds. "It's nice to buy clothes off the rack when they have my size in a lot of different colors—I don't have to just buy the one they have in my size."

Joe sees himself making Refuel a permanent part of his life. "For the first time in my life I feel like I've got a good program down—I could definitely stay here."

Best Tips

- **Cut down on alcohol.** "I used to drink almost every night; my wife and I would share a bottle of wine or I'd have a martini. Now, I don't drink during the week and it's definitely made a big change—in my weight, I'm sure, but also in my energy and sleep."
- **Check your carbs.** "Read a label and compare the serving suggestion to the quantities you're currently eating—it's shocking. Becoming aware of the makeup of foods really helped. I always thought a fruit salad would be a great choice, but it's not the smartest thing on a regular basis."
- **Sweat instead of snack.** "I usually find I'm hungry around 3:00 P.M., but instead of eating I'll use that time to work out. Then, we move up dinner to 5:00 instead of eating later."

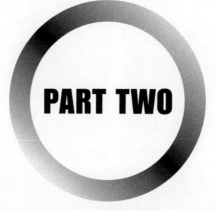

PART TWO

THE SOLUTION

**MASTER YOUR METABOLISM, LET WOMEN IN,
AND RELY ON THE RULES**

4

THREE QUIZZES

Do You Have Low T? Are You Fat? What Are Your 24-Day Goals?

I've studied thousands of men who have lost weight and kept it off. One thing they all share is that they measured their starting point. They knew their weight and they often measured their waist. They established goals, and they wrote them down, whether it was pounds, or notches on a belt, or completing an event like a local 5k, or something longer.

The quality of the starting data is key. That's where the Self-Assessment for Men (SAM) comes in, providing you with three quizzes to assess the numbers you need to know and leaving out the ones you don't. You don't have to do the research to find out which measurements are most important because I've done that for you.

THE MEASURE OF A MAN

Where do you stand in relation to the average American male? He's 23 pounds overweight and has a waistline of about 40 inches—5 full inches larger than the largest it should be. If you can relate, it's time to change. I'm going to show you how to lose weight and waist, once and for all. The goal is to shrink your waist so

that it's half your height or less. (Alternatively, you could get taller.) The playbook
is simple: make healthy behaviors so easy that it's easier to do them than to not
do them.

With SAM, I've created a way to measure your testosterone without a blood draw, a way to find out why you're overweight, and a way
to give you specific goals to hit. Tracking progress in an objective way
has another benefit. It's a little like having a deadline; you meet dead-
lines through full engagement and commitment.

SAM'S BENEFITS TO YOU

- **SAM will give you an accurate picture of your starting point in key metabolic,
  physical, and medical areas—no needle poking, sweating, or coughing required.**
  Anything that gets you to start thinking more seriously about your health is
  something good. Answer the quiz questions and use them for personal assessment, for tracking progress, and for a conversation starter with your doctor. If,
  in addition to SAM, you would like to have blood tests, go to www.drjohnlapuma
  .com to find an appropriate laboratory and testing site, or ask your doctor for
  the test.
- **SAM will help you measure your progress in three areas: testosterone, weight-gain
  factors, and milestones.** You can use Part 3 to reassess your milestones on day
  25. And you can take the quiz again every twenty-five days to raise your awareness and keep track of changes in your body.
- **You'll benefit from a little healthy competition.** Throughout the quizzes, when ap-
  plicable, you'll discover how other men have scored. Don't worry about how you
  will score against them. This isn't an arm-wrestling competition on the Jumbo-
  Tron; it's a discreet way for you to stir those competitive juices in the name of
  self-improvement. Knowing where you stand in relation to other men will give
  you the impetus to improve or to sustain your numbers.

You can also take parts of this quiz online, at www.drjohnlapuma
.com, where you'll be able to get personalized feedback and compare
your score with those of other men who have taken this test.

HOW TO USE SAM

Here are the three parts that constitute SAM:

I. **Do You Have Low T?** SAM-Testosterone (SAM-T) tells you your approximate testosterone level and whether you should consider getting a blood test to see if you need specialized treatment.

II. **Are You Fat?** SAM-Action (SAM-A) indicates which factors are causing excess weight gain and putting you at risk for or causing metabolic syndrome (waist, weight, cholesterol, high blood sugar, high blood pressure, high blood fats) and heart disease (from artery clogging to angina to stent city).

III. **What Are Your 24-Day Goals?** SAM-Goals (SAM-G) helps you set goals for Refueling and lets you compare them with those other guys who once were where you are now.

PART I. DO YOU HAVE LOW T?

SAM-T–Approximate Serum Testosterone Level

You will need a tape measure, a scale, a mirror, and a calculator. Following the quiz, you'll see why each question and measurement is included, and then you'll get your score. Scores are most accurate for men not undergoing testosterone replacement therapy.

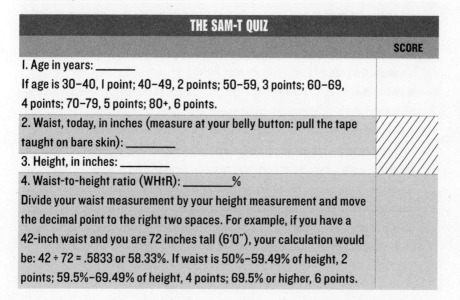

THE SAM-T QUIZ	SCORE
I. Age in years: _____ If age is 30–40, I point; 40–49, 2 points; 50–59, 3 points; 60–69, 4 points; 70–79, 5 points; 80+, 6 points.	
2. Waist, today, in inches (measure at your belly button: pull the tape taught on bare skin): _____	
3. Height, in inches: _____	
4. Waist-to-height ratio (WHtR): _____% Divide your waist measurement by your height measurement and move the decimal point to the right two spaces. For example, if you have a 42-inch waist and you are 72 inches tall (6'0"), your calculation would be: 42 ÷ 72 = .5833 or 58.33%. If waist is 50%–59.49% of height, 2 points; 59.5%–69.49% of height, 4 points; 69.5% or higher, 6 points.	

THE SAM-T QUIZ (continued)	SCORE
5. If over 60 years of age, have you had a hip or bone fracture since then? (2 points if yes.)	
6. Have you been told by a doctor that you have pre-diabetes or diabetes, or do you take diabetes medicine? (I point if yes.)	
7. Have you been told by a doctor that you have high cholesterol, or do you take high-cholesterol medicine? (I point if yes.)	
8. Have you been told by a doctor that you have high triglycerides, or do you take high triglyceride medicine? (I point if yes.)	
9. Have you been told by a doctor that you have pre-high blood pressure, or high blood pressure, or do you take high blood pressure medicine? (I point if yes.)	
10. Have you been told by a doctor that you have osteoporosis? (I point if yes.)	
Total:	

I. **Age:** After the age of 30, testosterone levels typically begin to decline at the rate of about I percent per year. This is what's considered natural decline, and we men can accept that, to a point.

What's not natural is for your testosterone to be consistently and massively depleted by way of aromatase. Your belly fat and the cells that connect your belly-fat cells to one another do that, every day. This testosterone depletion is driven not by age but by what you eat and how much abdominal fat you cart around. That's the fat on the inside. Fat on the outside equals love handles, which are easier to grab and not toxic. Except, maybe, to your swagger.

2–4.**Waist-to-height ratio (WHtR):** In 2010, Australian researchers noted an uncertainty about which physical measurement best predicted declining testosterone levels in men. Was it BMI? Waist circumference? Or waist-to-height ratio?

The answer they came up with surprised a lot of people: WHtR proved to be the best single predictor of both free testosterone and total testosterone levels. A healthy WHtR is one that's 50 percent or less. Here's a simple rule to help you remember this: your waist circumference should be less than half your height. So if you are 5'10" (70 inches), your waist measurement should be 35 inches or less—in which case, your waist would be exactly 50 percent of your height.

ABOUT BMI

Body mass index (BMI) is a widely adopted measure of overweight and obesity. It's one way to determine if you're at an unhealthy weight for your height. You should know your BMI because that's one route to a discussion with your doctor about what and how to eat. You can visit www.drjohnlapuma.com for a BMI calculator or you can calculate it yourself:

$$BMI = \frac{\text{your weight in pounds}}{\text{your height in inches} \times 703}$$

BMI isn't perfect, however. It overestimates body fat in athletes and others who have a muscular build, and it underestimates body fat in older persons and others who have lost muscle. It doesn't take a person's frame into account—and some people actually *are* big boned.

BMI presents problems especially for men who gain weight in their middle, where it is most toxic. For this reason, I prefer waist-to-height ratio over BMI. WHtR tells you what you really need to know: how much fat you're storing in your abdominal cavity.

Waist circumference by itself is just as powerful an indicator, and it predicts diabetes independently of BMI. That is, a waist measure of 35 inches or greater makes you 2.4 times more likely to develop diabetes; a waist of 40 inches or greater makes you 7.6 times as likely.

MAN MEMO

Do you know why some older guys seem to have a tight abdomen even though it's huge? That's because it's tightly packed with visceral fat, converting testosterone into estrogen, shrinking the testes, and making it harder to build muscle and increase metabolism. That's why.

5. **Hip or bone fracture:** Research published in the *Archives of Internal Medicine* revealed that the risk of fracture is significantly increased in men with reduced testosterone levels. This is true even after researchers adjusted for other major risk factors of age, bone density, fracture history, smoking status, and calcium intake. Major hits from professional football excluded.

6. **Pre-diabetes or diabetes, or on diabetes medication:** The American Diabetes Association says that a man with type-2 diabetes is twice as likely to suffer from low testosterone as a man without diabetes. A meta-analysis of over thirty-five studies published in the *International Journal of Andrology* confirmed this, finding that type-2 diabetes had a consistent, proven, and independent link to low testosterone.

   Low T appears before full-blown diabetes develops. Researchers writing in the journal *Diabetes Care* described how men with low T were twice as insulin resistant as men with healthy levels of testosterone. When you are insulin resistant, the levels of insulin and glucose in your blood are too high, putting you just about one Cinnabon away from developing pre-diabetes or diabetes.

   Like diabetes, insulin resistance runs along a spectrum. You can be pre-diabetic without knowing it. Usually, there are no signs, but if you develop dark, velvety patches of skin (called acanthosis nigricans) on your knees, knuckles, armpits, elbows, or back of the neck, get your fasting blood sugar and insulin checked—pronto. The patches are caused by insulin levels that are too high. In fact, if you are overweight or obese, you should be screened for diabetes; people with pre-diabetes often develop full-blown diabetes within ten years.

> ## DO YOU HAVE PRE-DIABETES?
> The CDC estimates that 35 percent of Americans aged 20 and over and 50 percent aged 65 and over are pre-diabetic; there are ways to tell if you're among that group.
>
> A fasting glucose level of 100 to 125 mg/dL indicates pre-diabetes (if measured twice, on different days), as does a hemoglobin A1c level of 5.7 to 6.4 percent. If you have high triglycerides or high cholesterol, or high blood pressure, or a waist circumference of over 40 inches, test your blood sugar level or glycohemoglobin or both, and get a testosterone test if your score is high on SAM-T. Don't wait a minute longer before starting to Refuel™.

7-8. **High cholesterol or high triglycerides:** Low testosterone levels are associated with increased risk for dyslipidemia. This condition means "screwy fat functions": you have high total cholesterol (TC) or low-density lipoprotein (LDL) or triglycerides (TG), or low high-density lipoprotein (HDL). If you have a four-pack of lipid issues, you give the plaque in your bloodstream a VIP pass to your arterial walls; and with atherosclerosis comes increased risk for heart attack, not to mention erectile dysfunction.

It's worth noting that high cholesterol is not just a malady affecting older men. In February 2011, German researchers reported that men ages 20 to 39 with low T levels had the highest risk of dyslipidemia. Other research, this time in Norway, evaluated the correlation of testosterone and cholesterol in 1,274 men and found the nefarious pairing of high TG and low HDL connected to significantly lowered levels of testosterone.

> ## MAN MEMO
>
> Testosterone production actually begins in the brain. Your hypothalamus sends a signal to your pituitary gland, which then produces follicle-stimulating hormone (FSH) and luteinizing hormone (LH). The LH hits the blood highway and takes it straight down to your testes to deliver an important message: "Guys, it's time to make some testosterone." The testes then get to work by producing testosterone from cholesterol.
>
> This does not mean that the more cholesterol you eat, the more T you'll make. Your liver makes all the cholesterol you need. Men who lose the gut probably have better testicular responsiveness (say it three times fast) and higher T levels as a result.

9. **Pre-hypertension, or high blood pressure, or taking high blood pressure medication:** Men with prehypertension (systolic from 120 to 139, or diastolic 80 to 89) are 3.5 times more likely to suffer heart attacks than those with normal blood pressures. According to the CDC, nearly 30 percent of American adults ages 20 and older are pre-hypertensive.

    Researchers reporting in the *European Journal of Endocrinology* had this to say about blood pressure and T: "men with hypertension had lower levels of total and free testosterone." Their findings were consistent with other research that had connected low testosterone with other heart disease risk factors.

    Additional research in 2012 revealed a deeper role for testosterone and the blood vessels. In their article "Association of Testosterone Levels with Endothelial Function in Men," published in *Arteriosclerosis, Thrombosis, and Vascular Biology*, researchers found that low testosterone is associated with impaired endothelial function. The endothelium is a thin layer of cells inside the arteries that helps them fend off the damage caused by LDL. When both endothelial dysfunction and high blood pressure are present, they can be a deadly duo, and low T has a proven link to both conditions.

> **MAN MEMO**
>
> Do you have white-coat hypertension? This is the high blood pressure brought about by the jitters associated with a visit to the doctor's office. The most precise way to know if this is the cause of your high blood pressure is to compare the doctor's measurement with a 24-hour monitoring system at home. But even if the sight of a white coat has spiked your blood pressure, the high results shouldn't be written off: Italian researchers found that subjects with white-coat hypertension were at greater risk for developing the real affliction down the road.
>
> I ask my patients with high blood pressure to measure their blood pressure twice daily at home in each arm—in the morning and evening—instead of using a 24-hour monitor. This is easier, it's less costly, and it clues them in on what is happening in their bodies. Knowing your blood pressure is more important than knowing your golf handicap—high blood pressure quadruples the risk of stroke. I like many of the easy, do-it-yourself blood pressure machines with digital read-outs and memories; some now also upload the results to the Web.

10. **Osteoporosis:** This condition of thinning and weakened bones is often misunderstood as solely a "woman's disease," despite the fact that millions of American men are afflicted by it each year. In fact, one-third of all osteoporotic bone fractures occur in men, and death after a hip fracture—one of the most serious risks of osteoporosis—is more common in men than in women.

    The risk for thinning bones naturally increases with age, but there are other factors that can speed the process; for example, steroid medications, excessive drinking, smoking, and low levels of testosterone. Research shows men with low testosterone levels are more likely to develop osteoporosis. In particular, a study of 2,447 men over the age of 65 found that those with low total T were more than three times as likely to experience rapid bone loss in the hips as those with normal levels.

    To help prevent osteoporosis from developing, ensure that your sex hormone levels are healthy and use your bones: walk, jog, weight train, do resistance exercises, garden, prune trees. All of these activities demand that your muscles and bones work against gravity—especially lifting weights while gardening.

MYTH: MY MUSCLES ARE WEAK BECAUSE I'M OVERWEIGHT.

Highly unlikely. Overweight men and women have to carry around extra pounds, by definition, and that builds up the big muscles—the glutes, quads, lower back. Most overweight people are quite strong, and the load bearing is also reflected in strong bones. But that's all the more reason to be concerned if you have osteoporosis. Overweight guys over 60 years old who have osteoporosis have very low testosterone levels until proven otherwise. That's true no matter what your musculature.

Understanding Your SAM-T Score

Total possible points: 19

Very low testosterone: 14 to 19

In general, this range suggests that your T levels may have undergone a moderate to severe decline and you've experienced significant metabolic or biological disturbances due to diminished testosterone.

Low testosterone: 8 to 13

In general, this range suggests that your T levels may have undergone a mild to moderate decline and you've experienced some metabolic or biological disturbances due to diminished testosterone.

Acceptable testosterone: 7 or less

In general, this range suggests that your T levels are healthy and you've experienced little to no metabolic or biological disturbances due to diminished testosterone.

The SAM-T score offers a general assessment of testosterone levels and will not be accurate for everyone. This quiz should not replace the tests administered by the medical professional but, rather, incentivize you to seek out further testing, should you need or want it. Look for laboratory options at www.drjohnlapuma.com.

More Reasons to Care About Your T Level, Now and in the Future

Even if you scored in the range of acceptable testosterone levels, you may still have symptoms that could indicate your T is teetering on decline. The following are general symptoms associated with low T in men with excess abdominal fat:

Low libido
Lack of initiative, assertiveness,
    and drive
Fatigue
Decreased sense of well-being and
    self-confidence
Depressed, irritable moods
Indecisiveness

Decreased mental sharpness
Lessened stamina and endurance
Loss of muscle mass, strength,
    and tone
Decline in morning erections
Decline in sexual ability
Sleep apnea

If you are experiencing any of these symptoms, Refuel will help you tackle them head-on. Men who used Refuel noted improvements in energy, mood, erectile function, mental acuity, confidence, and muscle mass and tone, and lost dangerous abdominal fat. In just 24 days.

There are other reasons you should care, as you probably know by now: low testosterone is a harbinger of serious medical conditions and other maladies. Here are some other ways in which low T could affect you:

Metabolically: When researchers in Boston, Massachusetts, put sixty men through a hormonal and metabolic evaluation, they found a strong link between low testosterone and lowered insulin sensitivity.

Ninety percent of the men with low T levels met the criteria for metabolic syndrome. Even though obesity may lower your testosterone levels, low T may also predispose you to visceral obesity, setting up a chicken-or-the-egg debate. The relationship is what's referred to as "bidirectional"—that is, each condition perpetuates the other. What matters more than the origin of the relationship is putting an end to it.

One thing is clear: lose your belly fat, and your testosterone levels will improve.

Medically: Low T is more than marketing hype—it has been linked to increased risk of diabetes, early death, heart disease, Alzheimer's disease, metabolic syndrome, and depression. What is the other serious medical condition linked with low testosterone? Erectile dysfunction (ED). Yet the relationship between erectile dysfunction and serious medical conditions isn't exactly what you would think.

It's not more testosterone that your body needs to fuel firm erections; it's silky smooth blood flow. When you're aroused, your brain triggers a surge of blood to the penis, which fills the thousands of blood vessels in the shaft and brings your sex soldier to full attention. If your circulation and blood flow are compromised, your erection will not be as strong as it could be. It's the low testosterone link to diminished blood flow—and diminished desire—that connects it to erectile dysfunction.

▶ MAN MEMO

You can promote proper blood flow through your body by making sure you have enough L-arginine. This important amino acid helps produce nitric oxide (NO), which acts like a "chill pill" for your blood vessels. That is, when NO is present, the blood vessels relax and open up, allowing the blood to pass through freely. Better blood flow is a boon for the entire body, your penis included, as good flow translates to stronger and longer erections.

Prime your body to produce NO by getting ample L-arginine into your diet by eating foods like nuts, seafood, beans, and eggs. Put some chill in your bowl with my Jamaican Two-Bean Veggie Soup (page 215).

The good news about erectile dysfunction is that it's not usually a psychological issue (although it could become one). The bad news is that it's an early warning sign for heart disease. You don't want to show up at the emergency room throwing up, with chest pressure and shortness of breath, surprised that you weigh 267 pounds when you thought you weighed 240, and just had trouble in bed, not trouble in the heart.

If you are experiencing ED, Refuel can help—57 percent of men on the program who could improve their erectile function have. However, you should see your physician and ask about having a cardiac stress test, now. They don't call ED an early warning sign for nothing.

Psychologically: Low testosterone can make a serious dent in your overall well-being, decreasing your initiative and energy and increasing your anxiety, irritability, and risk of depression. Men who are clinically depressed have lower T levels than men who are not depressed, and they have fewer orgasms and less desire. As a double whammy, some antidepressant medications cause weight gain. (See page 41 for a list.) Testosterone replacement therapy can help men who are both clinically depressed and testosterone deficient.

For most men, fortunately, low T doesn't mean serious mental illness or clinical testosterone deficiency, though. If abdominal fat has taken some of your testosterone and turned it into estrogen, you can help restore a normal T level and improve your mood, too. This doctor prescribes Refuel to boost your mood: nearly seven out of ten men who stick to the plan for 24 days report increased energy and improved mood.

▶ IS SYNTHETIC T FOR ME?

You may be wondering—if your T levels are low, why wouldn't you just take a testosterone supplement? You might want to, and if your doctor recommends it, you should consider it.

But here are some other considerations. First, most men don't have levels low enough to require medication, nor do they want to inject, rub on, or otherwise apply hormones. Second, supplementation comes with side effects, the most serious of which is that it turns off your natural T production; that is, your system recognizes that testosterone is coming from somewhere else, so it shuts down the factory. Third, other reported side effects are shrunken testes, reduced sperm count, acne, a high red blood cell count, gynecomastia (moobs), and prostate enlargement. Fourth, unless you are one of the 5 percent of men who actually need testosterone replacement, you probably can do it naturally with Refuel. Try it first and you'll see; you'll have none of the risks and all of the benefits.

A Natural Boost

There are several ways to increase your testosterone levels naturally. You will find them explained in this book.

For example, regular exercise can help you increase testosterone levels that are already at a normal level. Even watching your favorite team win a game elevates your testosterone levels, while losing that game decreases it. Succeeding the first day on Refuel will help raise your testosterone levels; every success does. And you can expect other benefits if you have very low or low T, and you raise it using Refuel.

Higher testosterone does the following for you:

Initiates the production of sperm by the testes

Enhances libido and sexual potency

Promotes the development of muscle mass, strength, and tone

Decreases body fat

Promotes increased bone mass

Stimulates the production of red blood cells by the bone marrow; these red blood cells carry oxygen to the body's cells

Increases metabolism by enhancing the conversion of the inactive thyroid hormone, T4, to the active thyroid hormone, T3, within the cells

Can reverse gynecomastia ("moobs")

The best way to verify your SAM-T score is to have a blood test for total testosterone level. You can also copy your SAM-T quiz results from this chapter or print out the quiz from www.drjohnlapuma.com, and then take it to your doctor and ask whether a testosterone blood test is appropriate. Or, find a testosterone and estrogen blood test on my website to quantify your blood level; once you have the results, bring them and a copy of the quiz to your doctor to discuss.

PART II. ARE YOU FAT? (SAM-A)

Sam-Action

This test of habits will help you determine what behavioral factors
are making you fat, unhealthy, or both. In this quiz, you focus on the
tangible details of your life and generate a true measure of where you
stand and what you need to fix.

Completing the quiz isn't hard and isn't a huge time investment. It
does require scoring. **Score a "1" for yes answers and a "0" for no
answers.** Take the quiz the day before you start the Refuel program,
and then again when you finish on day 25. At the end of the quiz, I
explain why each of the items is important.

THE SAM-A QUIZ			
DATES:	TODAY ___	DAY 25 ___	REFUEL RESULTS
1. I eat fast-food meals more than once a week.			58% of successful men decrease consumption of fast-food meals.
2. I eat potatoes in any form, or sauced, fried, breaded, or battered foods, every day.			
3. I eat quickly, without chewing my food 10 times per bite.			83% of men learn to put more chew in their food.
4. I drink soda, sweet tea, or fruit juices every day.			
5. I regularly heat or eat hot foods in plastic containers, including microwaveable containers.			
6. I don't take an omega-3 dietary supplement or medication, or eat cold-water fish at least three times weekly (see page 84).			

THE SAM-A QUIZ (continued)			
DATES:	TODAY _____	DAY 25 _____	REFUEL RESULTS
7. I don't take a vitamin D dietary supplement or medication, or get 10 minutes of direct sun without sunblock three times a week.			
8. I don't often wake from sleep feeling fully rested.			66% of men wake up feeling fully rested more often.
9. I take any of the following medicines (½ point for each): Insulin, Neurontin, Lyrica, Depakote, Lithium, Nardil, Remeron, Celexa, Prozac, Paxil, Zoloft, Elavil, Tofranil, Tenormin, Inderal, Clonidine, Thorazine, Haldol, Clozapine, Zyprexa, Seroquel, Risperadal, Diabinese, Glucotrol, Glynase, Actos, Avandia			
10. I don't take nutritional supplements or a multivitamin.			
11. I smoke or use tobacco.			
12. I work around or have regular (several times weekly) exposure to chemical pesticides, herbicides, fungicides, fumigants, insecticides, paints, dioxin, or other environmental toxins.			
13. I often feel stressed at work or school.			75% of men report less stress after 24 days.
14. I often feel stressed outside of work or school.			

> **MAN MEMO**
> Saltwater fish from cold waters are rich in monounsaturated and polyunsaturated fats, particularly omega-3 fatty acids. Herring, salmon, mackerel, and sardines are the best cold-water fish to eat.

Understanding Your SAM-A Score

Total possible points: 26.5

A score of 5 or less: you can easily overcome your barriers

A score of 6–10: you're in the middle of the pack, but you've been there before and we both know you can beat it

A score of 11+: you have some serious work to do; let's get started

1. **I eat fast-food meals more than once a week.** Fast (i.e., highly processed) food is the freeway to obesity. Consumption of fast foods strongly correlates to a bigger waist (I'm talking to you, buddy) and increases the risk of severe obesity, high triglycerides, and low HDL (aka healthy cholesterol). Eating fast food twice a week can add 10 extra pounds to your belly in a year. A diet heavy in fast food also doubles a person's chances of developing insulin resistance.

2. **I eat potatoes in any form, or sauced, fried, breaded, or battered foods, every day.** Potato chips lead the list of foods most likely to result in weight gain, according to a 2011 Harvard study. Potatoes in any preparation should be consumed in moderation; whether boiled, mashed, or fried, they were associated with weight gain over a four-year period. Potatoes are a high-glycemic food, which when eaten excessively has been associated with a greater risk of developing aggressive forms of prostate cancer.

   As for other fried foods, a study published in the *American Journal of Cardiology* found that consuming fried fish led to increases in blood pressure and compromised function in the left ventricle. That's the heart chamber you need to keep your blood pumping. Foods that are sauced, breaded, and batter-fried are typically coated with carbs and crap that disguise flavor and help you store fat. Dr. Frank Hu, professor of nutrition and epidemiology at Harvard, has said, "The idea that there are no 'good' or 'bad' foods is a myth that needs to be debunked."

3. **I eat quickly, without chewing my food 10 times per bite.** Men who eat rapidly—and the fastest-eating women still eat slower than the slowest men, on average—have twice the rate of diabetes as men who take the time to chew their food. Food should be tasted and savored, not inhaled.

4. **I drink soda, sweet tea, or fruit juices every day.** Extra sugar is a leading cause of overweight in men. Consuming sugar-sweetened beverages is also associated with a significantly elevated risk of type-2 diabetes in men and aggressive prostate cancer. It's been linked, too, to increased LDL, blood glucose, and markers of inflammation—all of which are frontline predictors of heart disease. Indeed, sugar-sweetened beverages pack on the pounds. Back away from the soda, sweet tea, and fruit juice, and no one will get hurt. For good, clean fun try Citrus Water (page 207).

5. **I regularly heat or eat hot foods in plastic containers, including microwaveable containers.** Foods should be hot in temperature or with spices, not with toxins. Heating food in plastic containers leaches endocrine disrupters out of the containers and into your food, especially food with fats, thereby increasing your exposure to estrogenic chemicals like phthalates and BPA. You can control this by avoiding such containers.

6. **I don't take an omega-3 dietary supplement or medication, or eat cold-water fish three times weekly.** Omega-3 fatty acids (by dietary supplement, prescription medication, or fish consumption) reduce the triglycerides in your blood, lower the inflammation, and for some people, improve heart health. Know your level; take an omega-3 home blood test.

7. **I don't take a vitamin D dietary supplement or medication, or get 10 minutes of direct sun without sunblock three times weekly.** Overweight men are more likely to have low levels of vitamin D, while higher levels of vitamin D mean higher levels of testosterone. Men with normal vitamin D levels (30 ng/ml or more) are much more likely to have normal testosterone levels, and a lower risk of heart disease. A vitamin D deficiency translates to impaired blood sugar regulation, failed DNA error correction, and increased risk of metabolic syndrome. It's easy to fix and important that you do so.

8. **I don't often wake from sleep feeling fully rested.** Sleep deprivation over the course of just one week can significantly reduce insulin sensitivity in men; even just one night of poor sleep can lead to increased food intake. Being short an hour of sleep a night is equivalent to pulling an all-nighter once a week. Short sleeping times have also been linked to impaired glucose metabolism and increased risk of type-2 diabetes and obesity. Sleep more (at least 7 and up to 9 hours), weigh less.

9. **I take any of the following medicines:** Insulin, Neurontin, Lyrica, Depakote, Lithium, Nardil, Remeron, SSRIs (Celexa, Prozac, Paxil, Zoloft), Tricyclics (Elavil, Tofranil), Tenormin, Inderal, Clonidine, Thorazine, Haldol, Clozapine, Zyprexa, Seroquel, Risperadal, Diabinese, Glucotrol, Glynase, Actos, Avandia. All of these

medications can cause weight gain. If you're taking one or more of them, ask your doctor if the medications could be contributing to your weight gain and if there's an alternative. Start Refuel to have a shot at lowering your dose.

10. **I don't take nutritional supplements or a multivitamin.** Multivitamin supplementation in men has been shown to improve mood, alertness, and overall sense of well-being, perhaps by way of correcting underlying nutritional deficiencies. The right multivitamin (see the Refuel Supplement Guide, starting on p. 164) will help supply vitamins and minerals that you aren't getting enough of in your diet.

11. **I smoke or use tobacco.** Do I really need to tell you why smoking is listed here? More people die from lung cancer than any other type of cancer, and men are more likely than women to die from it. Seriously, plan to stop smoking. Both smoking and smokeless tobacco cause heart attacks and strokes. Does smoking raise your testosterone levels? Yes, a little bit. But how does a little bit of lung cancer sound?

12. **I work around or have regular (several times weekly) exposure to chemical pesticides, herbicides, fungicides, fumigants, insecticides, paints, dioxin, or other environmental toxins.** Chronic exposure to environmental toxins has been linked to heart disease and endocrine disruption. Prolonged pesticide exposure also increases the risk for Parkinson's disease and other neurological disorders, as well as respiratory conditions. But most of all, these toxins screw up your production of testosterone and can alter secondary sex characteristics. They have been known to turn male frogs into mostly female ones. So, be a prince: get a mask, go organic in your gardening, buy paints low in volatile organic compounds (VOC), and stop using plastics whenever you can.

13–14. **I often feel stressed at work or school/I often feel stressed outside of work or school.** Chronic stress promotes chronic inflammation, which in turn can lead to atherosclerosis, a condition that underlies heart attack and heart failure. Sustained stress also bumps up your cortisol level, creating a constant fight-or-flight (stress) response. Sustained stress also spikes your insulin level, abdominal fat, and blood pressure. But you don't necessarily feel those things.

You do feel the everyday effects of stress: jaw clenching, frequent headaches, anxiety, chest pain, bowel problems, diminished sexual function, weight gain, frustration, insomnia, irritability, and fatigue, to name just a few. Chronic stress can't be resolved in a paragraph or two, but it can be improved with the right tools and changes, one step at a time. The result? Better energy, greater motivation, more self-confidence, higher drive, increased productivity, and maybe most important, a feeling of direction, excitement, and anticipation of what's ahead. Read on and find out how this happens.

PART III. WHAT ARE YOUR 24-DAY GOALS?

SAM-Goals (SAM-G)

Let's get physical. To know where you're going and set your goals, you create your Refuel profile with this third quiz. Check in with your body and ask yourself some tough questions: Are you really exercising that hard? You should be sweating. Are your muscles strong? You should be able to do at least 25 pushups—that's how many Michelle Obama can do, and Ellen DeGeneres can do 20. Real pushups, not "girl" pushups.

Take this quiz the day before you start your program, and then again the day after you finish, on day 25.

THE SAM-G QUIZ				
DATES:	TODAY'S SCORE _____	GOAL IN 25 DAYS	DAY 25 SCORE _____	REFUEL RESULTS
1. For every 5 days you deliberately exercise (walking, swimming, weights, playing a sport), how many days do you begin to sweat?				67% of men increase their number of sweat-producing workouts.
2. How many consecutive, full pushups (back and arms straight, chest lowered to fist-width from the floor, back up) can you do today?				67% of men increase the number of pushups they can do.
3. How many consecutive, full burpees (kick legs back to push up position, bring legs forward to squat, stand up, jump)?				42% of men increase their burpee count.

THE SAM-G QUIZ (continued)				
DATES:	TODAY'S SCORE ___	GOAL IN 25 DAYS	DAY 25 SCORE ___	REFUEL RESULTS
4. Enter your weight.				Refuel men lose an average of II pounds over 24 days (see chart on page 89).
5. Do you have hard morning erections once a week or more? Answer: Yes, sort of, no, not sure.				57% of men report more morning wood after 24 days.
On a scale of I to IO (I being none or poorest possible and IO being the maximum or best possible), how would you rate your:				
Libido (sex drive)				57% of men improve their sex drive.
Erectile ability				56% of men have better erections after 24 days.
General mood				75% of men notice improved mood.
Sleep quality				75% of men experience better sleep.
Energy level				89% of men have increased energy.
Muscle mass				75% of men feel their muscles are stronger and firmer.
Ability to concentrate				50% of men improve their concentration.

Once you've completed SAM-G for Day 1, take three photos. Two photos of yourself, taken today in a short-sleeve T-shirt and jeans with a belt, one photo looking straight at the camera, and one photo with your head turned 90 degrees to your right. The other photo should be of your scale, with your weight displayed. Put these images on your refrigerator, workstation, or wherever else you will see them daily.

Remember to take this quiz again on day 25, and every 25 days, to keep on the right track.

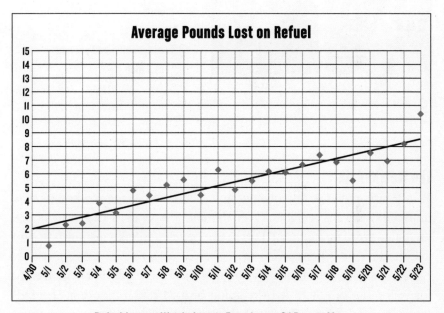

Refuel Average Weight Loss in Pounds over 24 Days in May:
11 pounds—nearly half a pound per day

READY, SET, GO!

So, what are you waiting for? Now that you've established a starting point and have your goals, it's time to begin dropping that belly fat and boosting your testosterone levels.

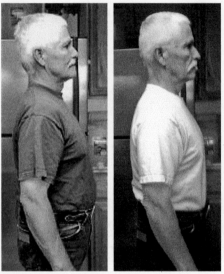

Day 1   Day 24

REFUEL SUCCESS

Name: **Tom P.**
Age: **61**
Weight Loss in 24 Days: **13 pounds**
Waist Loss: **1 inch**

The Weight Gain

Tom P. was never really a heavy guy. Then, as his age worked its way up, so too did his weight. "Over the last few years, I began to notice my pants were tighter. Or I'd go to the beach and take my shirt off and just think, *This is not good.*"

A mostly healthful diet and regular exercise habit had kept Tom fit for years, but one item kept nagging him: "I had a blood sugar reading come back high. The re-test three months later showed everything was okay, but diabetes is not something I want to get even close to—I know how terrible the disease is."

He never drank sugary drinks and he ate well-balanced meals, but snacks and high-carbohydrate sides were too often part of his diet. "The in-between times would get me—Fritos while I was golfing, bread and butter before dinner. And fried potatoes were often part of my breakfast."

Refuel came in sync with his motivation to create some changes in his life. "I was ready to make a commitment to improve my quality of life; to look better, feel better, and be healthier in general."

What Changed

Tom focused on carbohydrates when it came to modifying his diet. "I skipped bread, potatoes, and rice and I got my carbs from vegetables and fruits. The best part was that I found I was more satisfied by what I was eating and not as hungry."

He bought a scale with a feature that allowed him to input what he'd eaten each day. "I kept track of my calories and carbs for the first week or so, but then after that it came pretty easy and I basically knew what I should be eating."

The first challenge Tom encountered was the summer he spent in Montana. With a number of friendly neighbors all around him, Tom received numerous dinner and other invitations. "While here we're always getting together with different neighbors to have dinner, which of course means you're not cooking for yourself. I found the best strategy was to take only small portions of any dishes that weren't on the plan."

He did much better at home, where he received encouragement and sustained support from his partner. "It was nice to hear her say, 'You look great—it's really working.' "

What's Better Now

When Tom arrived in Montana for the summer, he had lost some weight and experienced clear and noticeable benefits. "My motivation and energy levels were just amazing," he says. "And my general well-being was better, too. It was the best summer I've had in years."

It helps, too, that the fit of his clothes had improved: two belt notches and tailored pants that are easy to put on marked a great start to his days. Tom says that even strangers have noticed. "One man said to me, 'You look great. You're *how* old?' "

Best Tips

- **Focus on one day at a time.** "I didn't think about doing something for the rest of my life; I just focused on what I needed to eat for that day—it's helpful to look at it that way."
- **Eat out less.** "Eating at home is the simplest way to know what you're really eating. But if you go out, it's possible to stick to the plan. For example, a breakfast I

ordered out was two eggs with sausage, no grits, and the biscuit to go, so I could
have it later with lunch."

- **Don't succumb to pressure.** "When you're eating at other people's houses, simply
  say, 'I'm trying to watch what I'm eating.' And just remember that you are the one
  who controls what you eat."

A PLATE FOR TWO

How to Bring Refuel into Your Home

Food, fitness, and relationships are all deeply intertwined. If your friends hit happy hour every night, it's more likely that you will, too. If your wife or significant other orders chili cheese fries or a slice of carrot cake the size of a toaster, you'll probably eat some—mostly, of course, because you're doing her a favor: "Share this with me; I can't possibly eat it all by myself." The problem is that you're not doing yourself a favor. Or her, really.

Weight gain is a proven side effect of love. Among married couples and long-term partners, the connection isn't just theoretical. In one of many studies, University of North Carolina at Chapel Hill researchers found that married or dating men and women who lived together two years or longer were more likely to be obese, and to be inactive and sedentary, together.

It's not just weight gain, but also the underlying habits that have proved to be contagious between spouses or partners. Researchers at Yale University School of Medicine and Duke University found that one person's habits had a "striking impact" on the other. Exercising, getting a flu shot or cholesterol screening, smoking, and drinking were all likely to be joint practices.

> **MAN MEMO**
> If your friend becomes obese, your chances of becoming obese increase by 57 percent—even if your friend is hundreds of miles away. Habits and influences transcend even distance.

This isn't simply a case of birds of a feather flock together but, rather, a side effect of equal parts comfort and routine. But what happens when that comfort has made you uncomfortable in your own body? When the routines and patterns of eating and other behaviors you've jointly fallen into have led to joint aches and pains, weight gain, and low energy? You've got to change your routine.

As you take steps to change your own routine with Refuel, it's likely you aren't doing so alone. The changes you make and will want to make will affect others in your home—and may even depend upon them. Refuel becomes all the more powerful when you know how to get the support you need.

THE REAL WORLD

To create a home environment that helps you establish and sustain Refueling, we have to look to the topic of communication (no leather couch required). The best way to demonstrate what works and what doesn't work is to examine real-life examples. Men who use Refuel offer insights into their experiences at home.

Top Encouraging Phrases from Women

ON APPEARANCE   • "I can tell you lost weight, especially from the side."
              • "Wow, you have lost so much weight."
              • "That Refuel sure is working."

Positive statements on appearance are productive and motivating; negative statements are counterproductive and can really take the wind out of your sails. Men on Refuel find that statements like these give them a little bit of swagger, and a lot of incentive to keep going. Tell your wife or significant other that you want to hear about the changes she sees, but not the ones she doesn't. Say, "To help me to stick to this plan, I would like it if you would tell me that I look good once in a while."

ON ENCOURAGEMENT
- "You can do it."
- "You look great."
- "You look healthy."
- "I'll do the shopping for any recipe you want to try."

If you've ever played sports, you know that a good pep talk can be a game changer. It doesn't have to be long-winded or come accompanied by a rump slap. In fact, it doesn't have to be a "talk"—just simple one-liners have proved enough to help Refueling men stay focused and on track.

Getting help with food shopping is a big-ticket item; even if she already picks up the groceries for the house, be appreciative of her offer because it means she's 100 percent on board and ready to kick in with help whenever and however she can. Say "Thanks for helping me make it easy to have the right foods in the house."

IN GENERAL
- "Your snoring has gotten better."
- "I don't want to lose you."
- "The kids really liked your dinner tonight."

If you live with your wife or significant other, she's not oblivious to the more or less visible symptoms of your weight gain. She sees your stress; she hears the tossing and turning or the snoring of disturbed sleep; she notices how you wrestle with the button closure on your pants or struggle to adjust your belt below your belly. She wants you to feel better and be healthier, but she also wants to hear less from you in the middle of the night, and more from you when you're relaxed and enjoying a nice meal at the end of the day.

Refuel men find the phrase "I don't want to lose you" helpful. I'm sorry if that's too much underbelly stuff for you, but it's the truth. I haven't met a male patient yet who doesn't want to hear that he's important to others. What most men don't want to hear is this same message delivered with a serving of criticism and an extra helping of guilt—or repeated ad infinitum, either. Remind her: empathy and kindness go a long way. Say "Thanks. My getting healthier is going to help everyone."

Least Helpful Phrases from Women

EXPRESSING DOUBT • "Are you going to go back to the way you were eating after the plan is done?"
• "This time, will it work?"
• "Are you sure this diet is healthy?"

According to Buddha's teachings, it's doubt that separates people. Let's just say that your significant other won't be helping you lose your Buddha belly if she doubts your commitment to the plan or its credibility. Assure her that the plan is based on science (see Bibliography, page 261) and has been proven in test groups to help men drop their belly fat, improve their sleep and erectile function, and boost their mood and energy.

Men on the Refuel plan find others' questioning their commitment to the program anything but helpful. Still, it may have given them something to prove: nearly two-thirds of the men who try Refuel lose more than 10 pounds in the 24 days. The best way to respond to those doubts is through action: you know what to do, and you just keep doing it. It doesn't hurt to say, "That's not exactly what I'd like to hear. I'd rather you offer to help than question my ability."

BEING JUDGMENTAL • "Don't lose too much weight."
                     • "Are you really going to eat that?"
                     • "I guess you're not going to exercise today."

Some guys on the plan expressed a "damned if I do, damned if I don't" predicament: their weight gain was criticized, but so were their efforts to do something about it. One way to take control of this topic is to share your weight-loss goals with your wife or significant other. When you take the SAM-A quiz, have her help you by counting your pushups or burpees, or just let her know what your goals are for day 25. If she's actively engaged in the process, she'll be more apt to offer encouragement. If you hear a judgmental remark like those above, try responding, "I'm trying to get healthy: saying something positive helps."

WHAT MAKES A MAN

Societal forces have to some extent been defining for you what it means to "eat like a man." Researchers tested various foods and habits to see how men and women rated them on a scale reflecting masculinity and femininity. Guess which items below were rated masculine and which were rated feminine:

Column A	Column B
Meat	Salad
Beer	Chicken
Smoking	Vegetarian foods
Triple-patty cheeseburger	Cooking
Doughnuts	Fruits
Pie	Vegetables
Fast food	Low-fat foods

It's pretty obvious: items from column A scored higher for masculinity and column B for femininity. The more important question to consider is, *Why* is it so obvious? How is it that men have become tethered to foods that are directly linked to poorer health, lower testosterone, diminished quality of life, and premature death?

Since women carry these same images of what masculine eating means, it's important that both of you shift your thinking.

The new masculinity is about fresh, strength-building foods and enhanced cooking skills. Being a modern man is being a healthy man. Modern men know the glory that is a perfectly roasted chicken: give it your best shot with my Roast Chicken with Lemon and Garlic Juices (page 219).

NEGATIVITY • "I have to cook something separately."
• "When do you get to start drinking again?"
• "When does the diet end?"

Refuel is a family-friendly plan from which everyone's health can benefit—a two-day low-carb, low-calorie eating method has proved effective for weight loss in women, too. Creating healthy food habits doesn't have to feel like running a three-legged race with the finish in opposite directions. Invite her to join you; it's one of the best ways to succeed. Say, "I'm trying to make a lifestyle change. I'd like you to do it with me."

> **HOT TIP**
If you're both eating to lose pounds, be careful: you can eat more than she can and lose weight. Instead of bragging about your weight loss, suggest that you set and meet individual goals (see page 87, SAM-G quiz).

Refuel isn't meant to send you straight to your man cave, hauling a brontosaurus bone. This plan is evolved eating, the sort that everyone can enjoy. The best way to counteract negativity is to include your family in the program.

As for drinking, the answer is simple: in Phase 3, you can have one glass of wine, a beer, or a cocktail twice a week. And you can stay on Phase 3 for life.

When it comes to the matter of when the diet will end, Refuel men discover that this is only an initial concern. Once men complete the 24-day program, the improvements are obvious: better sleep, improved mood, increased erectile function (for those who could improve), more muscle mass, and less belly fat. With such noticeable results comes full support from their families. Nearly every man states that he has no intention of reverting to old habits. As Joe F. said, "Refuel feels part of my life and is something I can stick with—I consider these permanent lifestyle changes."

Sharing this chapter with your wife or significant other might be a good move. Of course, not every weight- or health-related topic that comes up in conversation will be about Refuel; these exchanges can either be productive or be catalysts for verbal combat. Take a look at these highly recognizable conversations to see how to make them work for you.

What she says: *"Those pants are getting a little tight."*
What you hear: *"When are you going to get off your fat ass and do something about that beer belly?"*
What not to say to her: *"Why don't you mind your own freaking business?"*
What to say to her: *"Yeah, I could use some help."*

What she says: *"It's time for you to go get your physical with the doctor. How long has it been since the last one?" (See page 101 for when to get a physical.)*
What you hear: *The Wicked Witch or your mother scolding you.*
What not to say to her: *"It was two years and eight months, just like it was last week when you asked me."*
What to say to her: *"Yes, I know my health is important to you."*

What she says: *"Are you not attracted to me anymore? We haven't had sex in a month."*
What you hear: *"I've noticed you can't get it up, much."*
What not to say to her: *"Well, my mind has been on other things."*
What to say to her: *"Let's schedule a date and time for us."*

What she says: *"I picked up Caesar salad with chicken for myself and I got you the meat lover's pizza."*
What you hear: *"You will always be my big guy."*
What not to say to her: *"Who are you trying to look good for?"*
What to say to her: *"I'm trying to eat leaner; maybe the neighbors would like that pizza instead."*

What she says: *"Are you sure you really need to eat that whole bag of chips?"*

What you hear: *"You are not going to be doing anything I don't approve of."*

What not to say to her: *"Should I eat the pint of Haagen-Dazs instead? No, wait, you ate that last night."*

What to say to her: *"Some foods I can't have in the house or I'll eat them. Do me a favor and hide them. Don't buy them, even for the kids."*

What she says: *"I wish you were more in touch with your feelings about wanting to lose a few pounds."*

What you hear: *"I wish you were more like me."*

What not to say to her: *"I lost touch with my feelings when Oprah left network TV."*

What to say to her: *"I do want to lose a few pounds, but mostly I want to get stronger."*

What she says: *"You never talk about your feelings about your diabetes! Okay, you said it sucked, but that's not how I wanted you to tell me."*

What you hear: *"You're not telling me what I want to hear, and unless you guess what is in my mind, it doesn't count."*

What not to say: *"I am not an emoticon. If you want to hear about feelings, try staying home with me and the kids."*

What to say to her: *"I don't need to talk about it as much as I need help with establishing the right habits."*

AVOIDING HEALTH HAZARDS

The subject of doctors' visits is a big one, volcanic even. If you had a dollar for every time a woman in your life mentioned these necessities to you, you'd probably have enough money to buy that flat-screen TV you've wanted for the bathroom.

And it seems she always brings up the subject of doctors' appointments when you're least likely to want to talk about it: in the morning, at the end of the workday, or worse, during the World Series.

My advice is this: you might get tired of your wife, significant other, sister, daughter, or mom harassing you about not going to the doctor, but the truth is that you probably *aren't* getting the checkups you need. You can kick the can only so far down the road when it comes to your own health.

I hate to pull out the white coat, but it needs to be done: be a man and get yourself to the doctor for regular checkups. Your friends will still respect you, your family even more. There's nothing weak about wanting to maintain your physical form and functions; in fact, few things are manlier. Don't be that guy who gets the news as a sucker punch to the gut: "If we'd only caught it sooner."

Here are guidelines to schedule the recommended tests and screenings:

AGES 18–39

Blood Pressure: Every two years or annually if results reveal high (over 120/80) or low (below 90/60) blood pressure.

Cholesterol Screening: Annually if you have genetic risk for heart disease; otherwise, begin screening at age 35.

Diabetes Screening: Necessary now only if your waist circumference is 40 inches or more, your feelings of hunger and thirst are constant without reason (i.e., no change in diet or exercise regimen), or you have to pee frequently.

Physical Exam: Every two years.

Self-Exams: Every month. Check your skin for changing moles or other abnormalities; if it looks "funny" get it checked. Skin cancer is no joke. If you have a family history of testicular cancer, check your testes once a month, too: roll your fingers over the surface of each testicle, feeling for abnormalities. A hard pea-sized lump or an enlarged testicle should be checked by your doctor.

Sexually Transmitted Diseases (STDs): If you are sexually active with more than one partner or don't use a condom (not a doctor-recommended habit), get screened every six months for STDs, such as syphilis, chlamydia, and HIV.

Testosterone Screening: If you experience low sex drive, erectile dysfunction, or unusual levels of fatigue or depression, ask your doctor about getting a blood test.

AGES 40–49

Blood Pressure: As for ages 18–39.

Cholesterol Screening: Every five years, or more frequently if you've had abnormal results. No doctor's visit required (see page 15 for how to read your score).

Diabetes Screening: Annually beginning at age 45, or earlier if your waist circumference is 40 inches or more, your feelings of hunger and thirst are constant without reason (i.e., no change in diet or exercise regimen), or you have to pee frequently.

Physical Exam: Every two years.

Prostate Specific Antigen (PSA) Blood Test: Annually, beginning at age 45, if you have a family history of prostate cancer or you are African American; both are considered high-risk groups. An increase in PSA levels can indicate infection, enlargement, or cancer, and treatment is more effective and less invasive the earlier these conditions are caught.

Self-Exams: Every month. Check your skin for changing moles or other abnormalities.

Testosterone Screening: As for ages 18–39.

AGES 50–64

Blood Pressure: As for prior ages.

Cholesterol Screening: As for prior ages.

Colon Cancer Screening: Every five to ten years or annually if you have a family history of colorectal polyps or cancer. Men get more colorectal cancer than women.

Diabetes Screening: As for ages 40–49.

Physical Exam: Annually.

Prostate Specific Antigen (PSA) Blood Test: As for ages 40–49.

Self-Exams: Every month. Check your skin for changing moles or other abnormalities.

Testosterone Screening: As for prior ages.

AGES 65 AND OLDER

Abdominal Aortic Aneurysm Screening: A one-time screening necessary only if you are between the ages of 65 and 75 and have ever smoked. Recommended too if you have a family history of aortic aneurysm, especially in your father or brother.

Blood Pressure: As for prior ages.

Cholesterol Screening: As for prior ages.

Colon Cancer Screening: Every five to ten years until age 75, or annually if you have a family history of colorectal polyps or cancer.

Diabetes Screening: Every three years. Or more frequently if your waist circumference is 40 inches or more, your feelings of hunger and thirst are constant without reason (i.e., no change in diet or exercise regimen), or you have to pee frequently.

Hearing Exam: Annually.

Physical Exam: Annually.

Prostate Specific Antigen (PSA) Blood Test: Every year until age 70. An increase in PSA levels can indicate infection, enlargement, or cancer, and treatment is more effective and less invasive the earlier these conditions are caught.

Self-Exams: Every month. Check your skin for changing moles or other abnormalities.

Testosterone Screening: As for prior ages.

6

THE FIVE COMMANDMENTS FOR GETTING IT UP AND DROPPING THE GUT

When it comes to getting it up and losing your gut, action overrides information. So as you get ready to start the 24-Day Plan, here's an important point: don't get too wrapped up in the details. Follow the dos and don'ts for each phase and you will be successful, whether you know what a xenoestrogen is or not. When in doubt, return to these Five Refuel Commandments. These are as constant as the North Star, and they will never steer you wrong. Learn them and refer to them often as you progress through the plan:

THE FIVE REFUEL COMMANDMENTS

1. **Do not eat foods you can crumple or crush.** Skip potato chips, hamburger buns, squishy bread, pretzels, and so on. These foods weaken muscles, zap energy, spike insulin, and make you store fat. No cheating—being able to crush a zucchini or an apple with a hammer does not count.
2. **Eat primarily undisguised lean protein and strong vegetables.** "Undisguised" means not sauced, dressed, breaded, coated, battered, or otherwise masked. Strong vegetables, like broccoli and kale, are those that boost your immunity and make you physically stronger.

3. **Eat only small amounts of grains, starches, sweets, dried fruits, and full-fat dairy, and tart up your carbs.** Any grain, pasta, or rice should get, at minimum, a sprinkle of vinegar, lemon, or lime. Bread should get mustard or salsa. Acidic foods lower the glycemic index of refined carbs, improve insulin response, and slow the rate at which carbs are stored as belly fat. Less belly fat means more testosterone for your body to use for muscle building and fat burning.
4. **Only use a 6-inch plate for meals at home.** This simple step will reduce your food consumption by 20 percent. You probably won't even notice the difference, except that your plate will be full when you start, and you'll eat with more pleasure because of it.
5. **Drink 3 liters of filtered (when possible) water with citrus juice daily.** Drink more water. You know why.

THREE LITERS OF WATER, SIX DIFFERENT WAYS

Exactly how much water is 3 liters? Here are a few different ways to look at the quantity (feel free to drink from the vessel of your choice):

- $6\frac{1}{2}$ 1-pint Mason jars
- 68 shot glasses
- $\frac{3}{4}$ of a gallon jug
- $8\frac{1}{2}$ large coffee mugs
- 4 27-ounce Klean Kanteens
- $6\frac{1}{2}$ American pint glasses

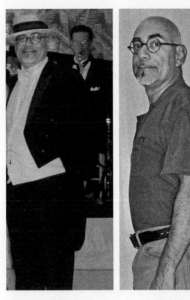

Day I   Day 24

REFUEL SUCCESS
Name: **Jim G.**
Age: **61**
Weight Loss in 24 Days: **12 pounds**
Waist Loss: **4 inches**

The Weight Gain

Over a four-year period, Jim G. experienced two big changes in his life: an elbow injury that put an end to his regular tennis matches and a new job assignment. The injury was a blow, but the new job as an elementary-school psychologist dealt an even bigger blow to his weight. "I was in a position now where I was eating a lot of school lunches, which are about as heavy in crappy carbs as you can get."

He had never had weight problems, but the combination of a lot of bad food and little exercise took its toll. "I gained about 15 to 18 pounds over four years."

A favorite suit for Fiesta, the yearly celebration of Spanish culture in Santa Barbara, California, gave him an obvious sign of what had taken place. "I wear this Fiesta outfit every year—and I put it on last year and it was really tight. I told my wife, 'I need to go on a diet.'"

What Changed

Jim credits an overall increased awareness for helping him make changes quickly. "I never really paid attention to what I was eating in the school lunches," he says. "But then I started noticing: mozzarella sticks with marinara sauce, nachos with cheese sauce . . . everything was high carb, high fat, and high calorie."

So he overhauled his lunches first. "I would stay up late or get up early to make sure I had my own food to eat." Despite its being the end of the school year, the busiest time for him, Jim felt sticking to the plan was simple. "I never had any problems following it."

He shifted other habits easily as well. "I started paying attention to what I was ordering at restaurants—looking for fish dishes with asparagus and salad. Always looking for protein and ways to eat more vegetables."

Jim also started reading labels, more to find out what was in what he was eating than to track it. "I didn't really count anything, but I did start to keep a mental calculation and focused more on what I wanted to eat and what I should limit. From the beginning I had success, so I didn't feel the need to log everything."

Drinking enough water throughout the day was a big change for him. "I was not drinking nearly the amount of water I should be. When I did, I realized I was not ever really hungry. I would not call this a diet because I was not obsessing about food."

What's Better Now

"I have more energy, I feel better, and I can exercise more," says Jim after completing 24 days of Refuel, which he plans to stay on. "The by-product is that people are commenting on how I look better and asking if I've lost weight. My face looks thinner—and my overall appearance does, too. And I moved a notch or two over in my belt so that's encouraging."

At 61, he says before starting Refuel he thought maybe the few pounds gained were just a part of getting older. But he was determined to wear his Fiesta outfit and to be able to perform in the events as he's done for years. The changes were worth it and they didn't disrupt his life: "It wasn't difficult. It's just as easy to make salmon and asparagus as it is to make pasta with meatballs."

The key for Jim was how he thought about what he was doing. "The beer gut has always been okay for guys, and we approach body image differently from women," he says. "I just made the decision that I really need to eat better, which sounds better than saying 'I'm going on a diet.'"

Best Tips

- **Focus on *can,* not *can't.*** "I really looked at this as a way to learn what I can eat, not what I can't. The general principles allowed me to personalize the plan to my tastes, but still while keeping everything within the guidelines."
- **Raise awareness.** "I liked not obsessing about food, but instead getting to know what I could eat and paying attention. On 50-gram days, I would typically eat eggs with ground turkey, salsa verde, and spinach for breakfast, a salad for lunch, and vegetables and chicken for dinner."

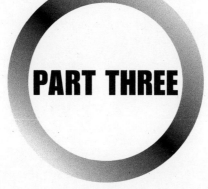

PART THREE

THE PROGRAM

24 DAYS TO GET YOUR MOJO BACK

REFUEL NUTS AND BOLTS

It's time to put Refuel into action. You'll follow three phases over the course of 24 days.

If you follow the plan as I've outlined it, you will be able to:

- Drop dangerous and disabling belly fat
- Pull the plug on the testosterone-estrogen conversion machine operating in your belly fat
- Feel more energetic, attractive, accomplished, and powerful
- Experience a refreshing clarity in your thinking
- See your muscle tissue firm up, shedding softness
- Sleep like a baby, wake like a man
- Have firmer erections and better sex drive
- Discover that you have productive new habits—automatic behaviors that you don't even have to think about when it comes to eating, exercising, sleeping
- Breathe better, stress less, be more productive

These are not fake promises from a fad diet: Refuel works, and it's helping change men's lives. I hope you'll be one of them.

THE THREE PHASES

Here are the three phases at a glance:

THE REFUEL PHASES		
PHASES	#DAYS	PURPOSE
Phase 1: Jumpstart	3	To act as the metabolic equivalent of the Polar Bear Plunge—promotes belly-fat loss from minute 1.
Phase 2: Boost Growth Hormone and Testosterone	14	To rebuild levels of growth hormone and testosterone, both of which stimulate muscle growth and maximize fat loss.
Phase 3: Maximize Energy	7	To make new habits permanent and enjoyable.

Before you begin day 1, let's review the three core elements of the program: eating, actions, and RE-UP. Implementation is more important than regurgitating the science behind the plan. Still, for the science and theory junkies in the crowd, this one's for you.

EATING
The 2/50 Technique

While following Refuel, you will apply what I call the 2/50 Technique: on two consecutive days of the week, you will eat up to 50 grams of carbs and about 1,000 calories a day. To jumpstart your metabolic engine (Phase 1), you will do this for three consecutive days. Then, for Phases 2 and 3, you will shift to following this 50 carbs/1,000 calorie pattern for two consecutive days of the week, alternating with days of moderate-carb (150–200 grams) consumption. Phase 3 will introduce some allowances that make long-term Refuel living easier and more pleasurable.

The focus on decreased highly refined carbs and sugar is not new, but here it's the cycling that works: going from two days of very low carbs to five days of low/moderate carbs, then back to two days of very low carbs, and so on. During the five-day period, you will realize how much better you feel eating foods that do not weigh you down (as so many processed and refined foods do) that you will want to keep doing that.

> **HOT TIP**
> If a food is a shade of white or brown, and it's in a package, it's been processed: sugary baked goods, fiberless breads, potato chips (technically canola oil yellow), pasta, and crackers have all been processed and are highly refined. Avoid these as often as possible. Naturally white foods, such as garlic, onions, shallots, and cauliflower, should be eaten freely and often. Cauliflower Popcorn (page 214) is one of my favorite sides—it might hit your top five list, too.

The 2/50 Technique is Refuel's trump card because this is what makes the plan sustainable. On those two days, your body burns the belly fat while you maintain muscle and feel energized.

This isn't the bodybuilder carb cycling you might have heard about. That's a low-carb, high-carb back-and-forth pattern used by bodybuilders for staying lean, especially before competitions. Best for bodybuilders, this method stores energy for massive workouts during the week. It's also not classic ketogenesis, a diet type that follows a 4:1 weight ratio of fat to protein/carbohydrate that is, by definition, very high fat (80 percent). Lastly, Refuel is not the Atkins or South Beach diet. The Atkins diet is meat-centric, and after its nearly zero low-carb initial phase, allows around 20 percent of calories from carbs; and of course, it's 24/7.

In Refuel, the focus is on plant foods as well as animal foods; it allows your total calories consumed to be between 30 and 40 percent carbs for five days out of seven, with just two days as very low carb; this way, you rebuild testosterone and stop its conversion to estrogen. Refuel's carb cycling gets you just close enough to ketosis near the end of day 2 that you burn fat first. But because you eat sensibly on days 3 through 7, you never bounce so high off the insulin charts that you want to tear the door off the refrigerator.

According to a 2010 study published in the *International Journal of Obesity*, the 2/50 Technique reduces fasting insulin (the amount of insulin in your blood after a fast) and improves insulin sensitivity, not just on the two days but up to an additional five days afterward. That's a full week during which your body is set to burn fat instead of store it.

And there's one more thing about the 2/50 Technique: you enjoy foods more when you haven't had much of them in a while, and when their portions are modest. Instead of inhaling your food, you have reason to savor it. Pleasure is the secret weapon in the program—absence makes the palate grow appreciative.

The key is to realize that it's the *quality* of the carb that matters, not just that it is a carb. Highly processed carbs won't efficiently satisfy your appetite, which makes it easy to overeat them; they fall short on nutrients and minerals, and they send your insulin production into overdrive, which leads to increased and nearly perpetual fat storage. On the other hand, high-quality carbohydrate sources such as vegetables are chock-full of nutrients and deliver a more balanced form of fuel. Whole fresh fruits and whole unprocessed grains are slightly lower on the quality scale but still acceptable.

If you eliminate sugar-sweetened beverages, fruit juices, and foods that you can crush in your hand (see page 103 if you need a reminder), you will have cut out nearly all calorie-dense, insulin-elevating, low-quality carbohydrates, including many with added sugars. On days you're not applying the 2/50 Technique, you eat a modest number of carbohydrates: 150 to 200 grams will further improve your insulin sensitivity, reduce your insulin resistance, and whittle away your body fat. And you'll look and feel better than when you eat more carbs than that.

You can use the Refuel carb chart on page 255 as a reference for many of the Refuel recommended foods. To check other food values, use any of these excellent resources online:

- www.calorieking.com
- http://ndb.nal.usda.gov/
- www.livestrong.com/thedailyplate
- www.myfitnesspal.com
- www. caloriecount.about.com
- www.carb-counter.net
- www.carbohydrate-counter.org

But Refuel is about a lot more than ditching the starches and the sugars; it's a full-plate, satisfying plan. Let's take a quick look at some other important components.

How to Fill Your Plate for Fat Loss, Fullness, and Flavor

EAT UNDISGUISED FOODS. Remember this important rule: your food should not be sauced, dressed, breaded, coated, battered, or otherwise masked when you get it. Not all sauces and dressings are bad—just ones to which you're not paying attention.

USE PROTEIN AS A PRIMARY COMPONENT OF MEALS. Protein, found predominantly in foods like fish, poultry, tofu, nuts, meats, eggs, and dairy, should be part of nearly every meal and eaten in ample amounts. I recommend natural food sources over engineered sources, such as protein powders, though these can work in a pinch. Food rich in protein needs to be front and center on your plate because it:

- Is slowly digested and broken down by your body, providing better and longer-lasting appetite satisfaction
- Provides amino acids, which support tissue growth, including muscle and hair
- Leads to greater weight loss
- Inhibits weight regain after weight loss
- Helps preserve and build lean muscle mass

Your goal is to select better sources of protein—those that have undergone minimal processing and have few or no chemical additives. Replace your favorite burger with a delicious Grilled Sirloin Steak and Asparagus (page 222). Drop the General Tso's chicken takeout and fill your kitchen with the aroma of freshly roasted, herb-filled whole chicken (see recipe, page 219). Swap bacon for simple homemade breakfast sausage (see recipe, page 225). Tofu and tempeh are also on the menu; more on these soy powerhouses later.

EAT THE STRONGEST VEGETABLES. "Strongest" vegetables are those that boost your immunity and/or make you physically stronger. These should be undisguised, too. Many of these vegetables are cruciferous, such as broccoli, cauliflower, and kale, but the sulfuric garlic bulb makes the cut, too (see full list, page 116). Cream of broccoli soup counts if you make it yourself.

▶ REFUEL CRUCIFEROUS VEGETABLES

Arugula	Collard greens	Mustard greens
Bok choy	Daikon radish	Radishes
Broccoli	Horseradish	Rapini (broccoli rabe)
Brussels sprouts	Kale	Rutabaga
Cabbage	Kohlrabi	Turnip
Cauliflower	Land cress	Watercress
Chinese cabbage		

EAT FATS, BUT BE SMART ABOUT STEAKS AND PROCESSED MEATS. Fat doesn't make you fat if you eat the right kinds and amounts. Sugar and starch do make you fat—for most Americans, anyway. But that's not a license to overeat cheese, butter, or whole milk. It is a license to maximize the flavor of food without masking its essence or sacrificing quality. That means you don't always opt for a nonfat yogurt or cheese or other less full-bodied version of foods you love. And you begin to read labels.

A little fat makes food tastes good, adds to satiety, helps you absorb nutrients more efficiently, and on 2/50 Technique days, is essential to keeping you satisfied. And saturated fat may not always adversely affect cardiovascular health (though it does raise cholesterol levels).

If saturated fat may not always cause metabolic syndrome and heart disease, what does? Foods that spike your blood sugar, raise your blood pressure, clog your arteries. We should be giving a closer look to high-sugar, high-starch foods with a high glycemic index (GI) and glycemic load (GL)—those that elevate blood-sugar levels based on how quickly they are digested and absorbed.

▶ MAN MEMO

Foods rank somewhere on the glycemic index (GI) based on how they affect the body's insulin and blood sugar levels. A carrot is a high GI food, but it has a low glycemic load (GL) because you have to eat a lot (i.e., pounds and pounds) of carrots to spike your blood sugar. You don't have to use this measure, but should you need to know: foods with a low GL are the ones you want.

Typically, high-GI and high-GL foods are highly processed sugary carbohydrates like cereal, bread, chips, and cookies. They cause inflammation, which probably leads to heart disease as well as disease elsewhere in your arteries, which connect to problems everywhere else: your brain, kidneys, liver, and gonads. They can also trigger the addiction center in overweight men's brains. Not good.

Sufficient research has been published to debunk the myth of saturated fat as the sole "bad guy" in heart disease and especially metabolic syndrome (about trans fat, there's little issue—it's bad). A meta-analysis published in the *American Journal of Clinical Nutrition* in April 2010 looked at over twenty recent major studies on fat and vascular diseases (including heart disease and stroke), and found no connection. All studies have biases, and this one may have as well. Still, convincing research exists to suggest that selective consumption is wise if you're trying to lose the gut and avoid excess calories.

Researchers with the Harvard School of Public Health tracked 121,000 people for up to twenty-eight years and found that a daily serving of red meat increased the risk of a premature death by around 12 percent. A daily dose of processed meats—one hot dog or two slices of bacon—increased the percentage of risk to 20 percent. Many red and processed meats like hot dogs are commonly grilled, so carcinogens created by high heat could account for the increase. Environmental toxins may also have a role—they get stored in fat, and red meats have a higher fat content than other sources of protein; more fat equals greater toxic exposure. Or the meats could have been served with a lot of starch and sugar, and few vegetables.

The bottom line is that while there are many forces at play, the takeaway from this study is this: When you eat meat, make it a healthier option (e.g., cooked well, without a lot of starch or sugar, and with serious vegetables). Eat moderate portions of red meat, and opt for the organic, grass-fed variety when you can. These organic sources are generally leaner, cleaner, and have lots of omega-3 fatty acids. They also have it over conventional beef in alpha-lipoic acid content—an antioxidant that helps your body fight damaging free radicals and has been shown to reduce blood sugar and improve insulin sensitivity in people with type-2 diabetes.

Here are the very best Refuel fatty foods:

- Avocados
- Nuts and their oils
- Coconut products
- Seeds and their oils (e.g., sesame, canola, hemp)
- Olives and olive oil

> ## MAN MEMO
> Go nuts before a meal—eat 19 pistachios, 10 almonds, or 4 walnut halves (about 65 calories' worth) 25 minutes before a meal, and you'll trigger release of the hormone cholecystokinin from your small intestine. That's a good thing: my friends Drs. Michael Roizen and Mehmet Oz called this phenomenon the tongue-twister "crucial craving killer," and that's what it does: it tells your stomach not to rush digestion, keeping you fuller longer.

Raise Your Glass (of Citrus Water)

Cutting out sugar-sweetened beverages (SSB) is one of the simplest ways to reduce your sugar and carbohydrate consumption. You should replace SSBs with citrus water (#SSBSuck).

There are dozens of reasons to drink enough water during the day. Number one reason: water keeps you alive. You've probably heard it said that the body could survive weeks without food, but only a few days without water. This is not a myth. Just like a neglected houseplant, we wilt and weaken without proper hydration. In the absence of sufficient water, your cells can't reproduce, detoxify, metabolize, or grow. So, drink three liters a day to keep all these functions operating optimally as well as to satisfy thirst, which is often mistaken for hunger. Dr. Sanjay Gupta notes, "The brain isn't very good at telling the difference."

To give hydration a kick, drink citrus water. When water has flavor, you value it more—it actually feels like you're drinking something. In addition, synephrine, an organic compound found in the rind and juice of citrus fruits, especially tangerines and sour oranges, accelerates metabolism. Citrus's vitamin C also helps to boost production of growth hormone, amazingly. If you don't like citrus fruits, a good substitute is zinger water, made with hibiscus blossoms. You'll find the recipes for Citrus Water and its variant, Zinger Water, on pages 207–8. They can be stored in the refrigerator for up to two days.

> **MAN MEMO**
>
> Hibiscus has one of the highest antioxidant capacities of any plant on the planet, and it can knock inflammation back where it belongs. Hibiscus goes by many names: red sorrel, red tea, Jamaican sorrel, red zinger, roselle: its scientific name is *Hibiscus sabdariffa.*

Get into the habit of carrying around a stainless-steel or nonreactive container of water. Aim to fill it with filtered water when you can; keep an eye out for places to refill when you're on the go. Restaurants with fountain drink service always have a water tap (ask for the lemons used for iced tea); restaurants will usually fill a bottle for free; use the drinking fountain or the tap in the bathroom in a pinch. Keep your water bottle nearby at all times and reach for it before you're thirsty and when you're hungry.

> **HOT TIP**
>
> Avoid weight-loss supplements with repeated reports of adverse effects. One product with additional synephrine, Stacker 2, has been linked to increased risk of stroke and heart attack.

ACTIONS
Motivation Overruled

Wouldn't it be great if motivation were something that could be borrowed or shared? You could ask that friend of yours, the one who is constantly on the go, always getting in a workout or heading out for a hike or triathlon (*does he even sleep?*): "Hey, buddy, I'm running low on motivation; could you lend me some of yours?"

It would also be great to win the lottery, but the odds of that happening are on the slim side. And they're not much better for some type of motivation-by-osmosis machine to be invented.

Yet so much of the discussion about losing weight focuses on motivation and willpower. There's an insistence on the need to "dig deep" or grind it out until you find your motivation. And that's really hard and pretty inefficient. If you're tired of digging, there's a better way. It all comes down to actions: what are your default actions, every day?

Most men's lives play out as a series of relatively predictable patterns and habits day to day (Navy SEALs and maybe POTUS excepted). As much as each day actually is a new beginning, or has the potential for one, can you think back to last week and recall what happened specifically on Monday versus Tuesday? Unless you experienced something out of the ordinary, probably not.

Think about it: you eat meals around the same time every day, walk by the same candy jar at work each day, drive past the same fast-food joints, drop off your clothes in the same place, and visit the same websites. This could explain why every day feels like Groundhog Day. But I'll show you how to turn the repetitive nature of your day into a Refuel advantage.

According to behavioral scientists, the key to creating change in your life is in identifying and tinkering with these patterns or habitual actions, not in trying to conjure up motivation or willpower. Change your habits, and you change the outcome.

> **MAN MEMO**
> Psychology researchers have suggested that it takes anywhere from twenty-one to sixty-six days to form a new habit. B. J. Fogg has shaken up those numbers with his concept of "3 tiny habits," which can be created in just five days by following his formula. I've modeled the Refuel Easiest Steps after this formula—find them on page 163.

Professor B. J. Fogg is a behavioral scientist noted for his ingenuity and focus on simplicity. A professor and researcher at Stanford University, Fogg has a very simple formula for how to change behavior.

Behavior = motivation + ability + trigger

Let's look at the parts to see how they come together to form a behavior:

1. **Motivation:** The fair-weather friend to action. Motivation can come from pleasure or pain—are you motivated to gain energy or to lose the gut?
2. **Ability:** The power to do something—the easier it is the better.
3. **Trigger:** The cue that kicks off an action. If you apply shaving cream to your face, you're going to shave—the application of the shaving cream in this case is the trigger.

You'll notice that motivation isn't entirely absent from the calculation, but you don't have to wait around for it to reach a high point to make new habits happen in your life. If you're reading this book, you can check off that part of the formula—consider yourself motivated.

Fogg's approach is to make the task so easy that with only basic ability and a built-in trigger or cue, your motivation can be low and you will still succeed. It's the "floss one tooth" (his brilliant example) approach: if you floss one tooth, it's easy. If you anchor the promise to floss one tooth to something you always do, you're more likely to do it. So your commitment is: "I will floss one tooth right after I brush my teeth tonight." (Naturally, if you floss one tooth, the other ones are right there . . . and you'll probably floss a few of them, too. But your commitment is to do just one—an easy promise to keep.)

One element is missing: reward. Yes, you get a reward for keeping your commitment. What is it? A look in the mirror and saying to yourself, "I'm awesome!"? A thumbs-up? A toothbrush that can Wi-Fi your brushstrokes to the cloud? Find a nonfood reward that you can give to yourself, and make sure you get it. It's part of the program.

Apply this formula to Refueling and create a new habit. For example, you want to drink 3 liters of citrus water a day. Simple, but not necessarily easy, so I'll make it easy to start: take one sip of water.

Using the trigger of pouring a cup of coffee or making a cup of tea, your commitment would look like this: "I will take one sip of water after I pour my coffee."

Your motivation might be moderate, but your ability to take one sip of water is sky-high. Chances are, you'll drink half the glass at least—and you should; drinking water in the morning boosts metabolism. As long as you pour your coffee, you'll take a sip of water. And your reward? Say out loud: "I am awesome!"

Here are more easy ways to trigger better choices:

1. Is there a regular route you drive that compels you to stop for fast food or junk food? → Go a different way.
2. Are there snacks in your cupboards or desk drawers that you reach for when starving? → Put new Refuel-approved snacks in those hot spots.
3. Do you want to work out in the morning, but for the life of you can't find a matching sock in the dim light of the A.M. (and you don't want to turn the light on and wake Sleeping Beauty)? → Set your workout clothes in the bathroom by the door the night before; change into them right after your morning pee.
4. Do you have to get all-you-can-eat wings with blue cheese dressing that pours out of a syrup jar every time you go to Wings-n-Things? → Drink a liter of citrus or hibiscus water and eat two hard-cooked eggs before you leave the house.

Plenty of behaviors are ingrained to the point of going unnoticed. Pull up to take a macro view, and you'll be able to see where you can make micro modifications. Make these small, tangible changes and you will begin to feel better. Give yourself rewards. Then, better will build upon better until you've created the foundation of the Refuel lifestyle.

Manufacturing Ability

Refuel aims to give you control of your food, but control is more about planning than about talent. You don't have to work to get good at eating right; you just have to reprogram your environment so it happens automatically. Here again the focus is not on chasing down your motivation, but on making it super-easy to do the healthy thing.

Psychologist Brian Wansink, who is the director of the Food and Brand Lab at Cornell University and the author of *Mindless Eating,* has spent decades studying consumption behaviors. He's found that everything from the size of the plates from which you eat, to the type of glasses you use, to where you sit can have a significant impact on how much you eat. Here, based on his research, are a few upfront actions that will amp up your ability and preparedness:

- Stock your kitchen with foods and supplies from the list beginning on page 197. This is the simplest way to ensure you're eating the right foods. If the wrong foods aren't there, you won't eat them.
- Eat meals on 6-inch plates. You will register the fullness of the plate, not the amount of food; a plate measurement includes the rim, which is not intended for more food. Six-inch plates are often sold as salad plates, or sometimes as luncheon plates. Look for new ones or check out garage or estate sales; carry a tape measure to check.
- Trade your short, wide drinking glasses for tall and narrow ones. The eye registers a vertical line as longer than a horizontal one. People will pour up to 30 percent more liquid into a short glass, yet they believe it's less than what they've poured into a tall glass. Drink everything but citrus and hibiscus water, coffee, and tea from tall, narrow glasses.
- Transfer bulk items you've bought into smaller containers.
- Portion your food—don't just grab a pint of ice cream or a 1-pound bag of almonds and start eating.
- Practice chewing each bite ten times. Men tend to eat more food and calories per minute than women. Slow down, and you will eat less food but still feel as full.

> ## ▶ MAN MEMO
> Your mouth is the first line of defense in good digestion. Poorly chewed food that's still in recognizable form—e.g., a barely gnawed-on bite of steak—is harder to digest, yields little pleasure, and sits like lead in your stomach, leading to indigestion. (#chew10)

RE-UP
The Rest, Exercise, and Unwind Protocol

Within each of the plan's phases, you'll see the phrase "RE-UP." When you see it, know that's where you'll turn for guidance on how to sleep, work out, and de-stress during that phase.

The Rest, Exercise, and Unwind protocol (RE-UP) is intended not just to maximize your belly fat loss but also to make you the best you can be all around. Improved well-being and quality of life is the whole package: eat right, exercise, sleep well, and decompress, and your daily life experience will be better.

In Chapter 3, I explained how the three components of RE-UP are part of a comprehensive approach to your heath, but let's recap:

Rest

You have to sleep, so you might as well get good at it—especially since the studies linking sleep and weight control continue to stack up, and many of them reveal that a lack of sleep takes a greater toll on men than on women.

A 2010 evaluation of the sleep habits of over 35,000 Japanese workers found that men were more profoundly affected by sleep deprivation than were women: less than six hours of sleep for men was significantly linked with weight gain and obesity. There was no such link shown in women. The gender differences have been apparent in other studies, too, revealing that less than seven hours leads to higher BMI in men. The bottom line: sleep times have a distinct effect on men, so make sure you're getting enough sleep.

But don't lose sleep over lost sleep. Instead, begin to implement simple strategies to get the most out of this critical rejuvenator. Getting between seven and nine hours of sleep a night will:

- Produce growth hormone, which will set the stage for muscle building, boost energy levels, and increase libido.
- Produce testosterone; like growth hormone, it is produced only at night, just before rapid-eye movement (REM) sleep, and gradually accumulates in your body.
- Help curb compulsive daytime snacking.
- Boost glucose tolerance and improve insulin sensitivity, keeping your diabetes risk low.
- Prevent dips in your testosterone levels.
- Improve your memory and cognitive abilities.

Exercise

In Refuel, we use modified high-intensity interval training (HIIT), a high-octane method designed to turn your body into a fat-burning engine. HIIT is a combination of two types of training: high-intensity training, which is about bursts of maximum or close to maximum effort; and interval training, which is about interspersing these intense bouts with periods of more moderate effort. In other words, you go hard and then you give yourself the chance to recover, then you go hard again.

There's simply no other type of training that works as efficiently to burn calories or build strength as quickly. HIIT also has a proven link to increased insulin sensitivity, and it works regardless of your fitness level—you determine what means "all-out" for you. Plus, since you'll only be exercising this way a maximum of 20 minutes at a time, you won't get bored.

You're going to do two types of HIIT:

1. **Cardio HIIT:** Designed to improve cardiovascular fitness and boost oxygen uptake. The more oxygen your cells and tissues use, the more calories you burn. Examples: walking, jogging, cycling, swimming, jumping rope, and climbing.
2. **Resistance HIIT:** Designed for functional fitness, meaning the movements will make you better at everyday actions. You'll perform exercises that engage multiple joints and muscles at the same time, such as pushing, pulling, jumping, and reaching; you'll do pushups, lunges, burpees, jumping jacks, and planks for an all-out short session and follow it with a brief rest period.

Within the workout instructions, you'll see the recommended intensity for the intervals. Rate your exercise intensity according to the following scale.

1. I'm a couch potato, literally.
2. I'm easily strolling.
3. I'm strolling still, but breathing a bit faster.
4. I can talk while exerting myself, and might be sweating a little.
5. I can still talk, but am starting to sweat and am definitely exerting.
6. I can still talk, most of the time.
7. I can still talk, but am somewhat out of breath; sweat drips into my eye.
8. I can grunt but not talk; cannot maintain long.
9. I might die if I push any harder.
10. I could have died, but didn't.

Here are the exercises you'll be using for resistance intervals; for cardio intervals, you already know how.

PUSHUP

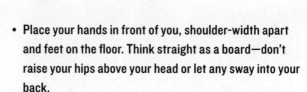

- Place your hands in front of you, shoulder-width apart and feet on the floor. Think straight as a board—don't raise your hips above your head or let any sway into your back.
- Inhale and lower your chest toward the floor, stopping when your elbows reach a 90-degree angle.
- Exhale and push yourself back up, keeping your legs and abdominals strong.

BURPEE

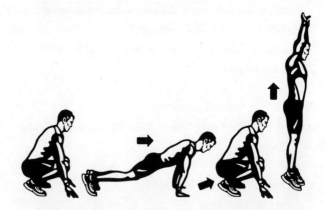

- Get into a low squat position and put your hands on the floor in front of you.
- Kick your feet back to pushup position.
- Return to squatting position, then jump straight up, off the ground.

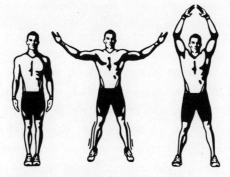

JUMPING JACK

- Stand up straight, arms at your sides.
- With a slight bend in your knees, swing your legs out and arms overhead simultaneously.
- Return your arms and legs to starting position.

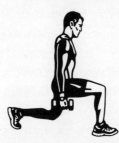

LUNGE

- Stand upright, then lunge forward with one leg.
- Lower your body by dropping your back knee toward the floor, making sure your front knee doesn't extend out beyond your toes.
- Return to starting position by standing up, pushing down through your front heel. Repeat on other side.

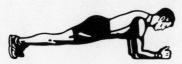

PLANK

- Lie facedown on the floor, with your knees touching. Put your forearms on the mat with your shoulders aligned directly over your elbows.
- Clasp your hands in front of you and assume a pushup position, keeping your forearms on the floor.
- Tighten your abs, and breathe evenly.
- Hold it.

Unwind

You probably don't need me to explain how stress affects your daily life: you feel it in your neck or back or you have tight, tense shoulders. You feel it in the indigestion that upsets your stomach and intestines, or the headaches, or the tightness in your chest. You also see it at work: chronic stress reduces your productivity and causes you to make mistakes. It makes you miss work and be less fully present when you are at work. Chronic stress makes you store more visceral fat, depresses your immune system, and leaves you vulnerable to colds, the flu, bronchitis, and injury—the last thing you need when you're stressed.

You can optimize your stress: you unwind and reboot not by fighting against stress or trying to remove it from your life, but by changing your mindset: you learn programmed responses to irritating situations, and make them work for you.

One of my favorite patients has an effective tactic for responding to a stress-inducing scenario. When someone says something to him that angers him, he says, "Thank you." If it's an email or a text, he writes "Thank you" and then saves it as a draft for a later, calmer response. Instead of perpetuating a tense situation and letting his blood boil (and blood pressure spike), he gives himself a millisecond to pause, and then if he likes, he responds. There's always a better way to respond than to do what reflexively comes to mind.

> **HOT TIP**
> Reserve swearing for a stubbed toe or jammed finger, not a stubborn relative. Letting off a few curse words has been shown to reduce feelings of physical pain.

During the three phases of Refuel, I give you breathing techniques and methods for simmering down, so to speak. Consider these more than anything else as productivity enhancers; you will, after all, be spending less time stewing and more time doing.

YOU CAN'T MANAGE WHAT YOU DON'T MEASURE

There are few things you can't track using a smartphone app or website these days—you can track package and pizza deliveries, flight schedules, muscle movements, budgets, brain waves, blood glucose levels, electrocardiograms . . . the list goes on. And most likely there's someone tracking that list.

You can use tech tools to your advantage in Refuel. But you don't have to go the electronic route; a simple notepad works, too. The latter was good enough for Ben Franklin, who diligently logged his adherence to thirteen virtues on a quest for moral perfection. To log your own food, print my Eating Day Book from www.drjohnlapuma .com, or copy the version on the next page for each day.

Thankfully, we're working with simple daily concepts here: what you eat, how often you work out, and how your body responds as it relates to your weight or waist circumference. Tracking what you eat is a form of self-monitoring, as it gives you a clear picture of your diet twice: (1) when you eat, and think about recording it; and (2) when you actually record it. A study from Kaiser Permanente's Center for Health Research analyzed the tracking habits of 1,700 people, and found that those who kept a food log lost double the amount of weight compared to those who didn't track.

For the 24 days of the plan, try tracking on for size. Perfection is not necessary, just effort. You should track three things:

1. **What you eat.** Most important, track 50 grams during Phase I and on other 50-gram days. On alternate days, be mindful of tracking. Or, if it's easier, just track for the entire 24 days.
2. **How much you've lost in pounds or waist circumference.** Weigh yourself on a scale every day; document the number. For a less data-driven measure, use your belt. Take notice of which notch you're using right now and make a mental note to keep an eye on it, daily.
3. **Duration and intensity of workouts.** Duration is simply time spent working out. You can break out warm-up time or include it as part of your total workout time; the level of detail is up to you. Use the intensity scale on page 125 to document your level of effort during each workout.

REFUEL

EATING DAY BOOK

Name:

Date:

Day (circle one): Monday Tuesday Wednesday Thursday Friday Saturday Sunday

Time of Day	Minutes Spent Eating	Meals/ Snacks/ Drinks—List each food	How Much of Each?	Hungry? Yes/No	Standing, Sitting, or Reclining?	Activity while eating?	Where are you eating?	Eating with whom?

Use this space to record your exercise—type, time, intensity, duration—for each day.

Technology has made tracking fascinating and cool, instead of a nuisance. I have found that texting men daily with specific action-oriented messages and asking them to text in their weight and intensity of exercise is very effective and helpful. If you'd like to try Refuel Texts too, check out www.drjohnlapuma.com.

TRACK THIS WAY—SAMPLE TOOLS					
	TRACKING	TOOL	ONLINE TRACKING	MOBILE APP	MONTHLY FEE
ALL-AROUND TOOLS					
Nike+ FuelBand	energy burned, steps, time, daily goal progress	water-resistant LED wristband	y	y	n
Jawbone Up	steps, distance, energy burned, pace, intensity level	water-resistant wristband	n	y	n
Runkeeper	cardio activities, distance, elevation, and time	none	y	y	n
Fitbit One	sleep, energy burned, steps taken	clip-on piece	y	y	n
BodyMedia	calories eaten and burned, sleep times	biceps armband	y	y	y
FOR WEIGHT CONTROL					
Bodytrace	weight, can log foods	Wi-Fi scale	y, wireless upload	n	y
Withings	weight, lean mass, fat mass	Wi-Fi scale	y, wireless upload	y	n
FitBit Aria	body weight, BMI, body fat	Wi-Fi scale	y, wireless upload	y	n

TRACK THIS WAY (continued)					
	TRACKING	**TOOL**	**ONLINE TRACKING**	**MOBILE APP**	**MONTHLY FEE**
FOR SLEEP MONITORING					
Lark	sleep patterns (also has silent vibration alarm)	wristband	n	y	y
Wakemate	dips and peaks in sleep cycle (has optimal wake point alarm)	wristband	y	y	n

y = yes, device does it; n = not done. Information current as of September 2013.

You can also use website apps designed for logging purposes, with no external tool needed. Here are some of the best (and free) available. All except for Worksmart Labs, which offers just apps, have website tracking and mobile apps:

www.LoseIt.com   www.fitday.com
Worksmart Labs apps, such as Noom   www.myfitnesspal.com
   and Calorific   www.fitocracy.com

These apps allow you to monitor your eating, workouts, and weight loss. For more excellent choices, sign up for the newsletter at www.drjohnlapuma.com.

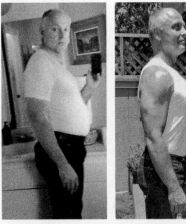

Day 1   Day 24

REFUEL SUCCESS

Name: **Wayne H.**
Age: **49**
Weight Loss in 24 Days: **11 pounds**
Waist Loss: **4 inches**

The Weight Gain

The initial weight gain began decades ago for Wayne. First, there was sympathy weight gain when his wife was pregnant, which turned into life-with-young-children weight gain. Then came more-business-travel-and-less-exercise weight gain. And so it went until Wayne H. was over 40 and 40 pounds overweight.

Wayne used to be an avid runner, but knee surgery and joint pain from extra weight took away the pleasure. He enjoyed dinners and conversation, but found sitting for too long uncomfortable—the pressure of his gut would contort his belt until it pushed sharply into his stomach.

A few years ago, Wayne decided on one major change: he would stop drinking soda. That step alone helped him drop about 10 pounds. "You drink sodas at restaurants where they refill your glass—and you're talking and you don't have any concept of how much you've had."

Still, there was more weight to be lost. He tried many programs that were about "just eating less—various versions of starvation diets." Nothing stuck.

What Changed

For Wayne, Refuel seemed different: "Two days a week required focus, but the other five days were just about being healthy and thinking moderation: eating a variety of foods, staying away from fried or high-sugar foods."

He began reading labels and increasing his awareness of foods. "It was eye opening: bananas, a favorite post-workout food, were surprisingly high in carbs." At restaurants, he started asking if they had nutritional guidelines. Meals he thought were healthy choices turned out to be anything but.

Wanye also stopped eating out so much. "I live alone and always thought it wasn't convenient to make dinner. I'd head out and get a burger or something just because I didn't feel like cooking, not because it's really what I wanted to eat." He stopped doing that. Now, he makes quick meals at home and cooks extra for leftovers: "I grill up enough food for three meals."

He also began walking to the grocery store, just ten minutes away on foot. "I would take one reusable bag and fill it—that was my shopping cart so I had to be selective. I'd pick up fresh vegetables, some chicken, and by the time I got to the aisles with all the garbage foods, I didn't have room. When I didn't bring them into my home, they weren't available to me to eat—pretty easy to avoid eating junk food that way."

Wayne never thought about the changes he made as just ways to lose weight. "I went into this thinking I was going to stay on the third phase for life—I wanted a comprehensive approach to changing my lifestyle, and I found it. I even made dinner for friends and told them, 'We're going to eat healthy tonight.' I grilled fillets and peppers and steamed some broccoli—everyone enjoyed the food, the flavors, and the textures. The bonus was that I was able to eat what I wanted and keep everyone else happy."

What's Better Now

Wayne has returned to running: "I lost weight and I can now run without pain." He can also sit without feeling uncomfortable: "There's no more pressure there from the weight of my stomach." Most surprisingly, he noted a significant difference with Refuel: he hasn't lost muscle mass, but gained it.

Plenty of people have commented and noticed the changes in Wayne. "I feel better all around."

Best Tips

- **Don't underestimate the power of hydration.** "I always thought I was hungry, but turns out I was not properly hydrated. I now grab a glass of water every hour or two—just eight ounces at a time until I've had three liters for the day. I feel more satisfied and have more energy."
- **Learn 50 grams for two days, but apply it all week.** "Once I started to get a sense of what 50 grams of carbs was, I would apply that times 3 for the other five days—just trying to eat about 50 grams of carbs each meal made it easy."

8

PHASE 1: JUMPSTART (3 DAYS)

When it comes to effort, you are more likely to make one if the rewards are clear and present. For this reason, the first three days of Refuel will reward you with accelerated weight loss—you put points on the board right away.

The science on behavior modification says that fast results are a strong predictor of success, and your gender gives you an advantage here. Researchers at the University of Copenhagen in Denmark found that the men in their study had the potential to drop more weight than did women during the first week of a plan, and that this upfront weight loss correlated with a significant increase in completion rates.

> **FAST STAT**
> Men who follow Refuel drop between 0 and 5.5 pounds (average 2.3) during Phase I.

In this initial phase, you promote a quick metabolic shift by eating 50 grams or fewer of carbs daily (see sidebar below). When you accomplish this by cutting out sugar or highly processed carbohydrate sources from your diet, you eliminate dramatic spikes in insulin, which otherwise would lead to increased fat storage and leptin resistance. The right carbs—minimally processed ones—are the ones you should eat.

▶ WALKING THE KETOSIS LINE

Refuel's two-day-per-week low-carb schedule helps trigger fat burning and mild diuresis (aka fluid loss), without sending you into full-blown ketosis. Complete ketosis comes from extreme eating: high fat, moderate protein, and very low carbs (fewer than 20 grams a day). This makes it too easy to stop a diet, in my opinion. If your brain does begin to use ketones (molecules that are formed when your body metabolizes fat, which are used for energy, expelled through the lungs, or excreted through urine) for energy, instead of stored carbs, you can sometimes feel the effects. Some people report bad breath at the end of day 2, or constipation, or a fuzzy brain feeling; all of these symptoms are real, and none of them should last more than a day. Unless you're constipated—and it's up to you to keep yourself hydrated and get enough fiber.

Since each individual's adaptation to low-carb eating may vary, if you find that you aren't thinking quite as clearly as you ordinarily do on the last half of day 2, check the rest of your diet for balance:

- Are you eating plenty of strongest vegetables (see list, page 116)?
- Are you hydrating yourself adequately?
- Are you exercising aerobically, too? You need to do cardio as well as resistance.
- Are you eating some healthy fat during the day? You need it for energy.
- Are you getting 10 grams of carbs, or 50? You should get up to 50 grams, and I prefer that you almost hit this number. It's more sustainable, and less dramatic. We don't need drama in our diet.

Liquid carbs should go on the chopping block first—sodas and juices especially, which have repeatedly proven to lead to increases in visceral fat. Soda consumption in men increases the risk for stroke and type-2 diabetes, as well. There's nothing good about sodas.

PHASE 1 DOS AND DON'TS

There are only a few key dos and don'ts for this phase; let's take a look at them.

Phase 1 Dos

1. **Eat up to a total of 50 grams of carbs each day.** If you do one thing only, do this. Carbs are in fruits, vegetables, grains, dairy, legumes, nuts, breading, drinks, sweets, sauces, and dressings, so keep these in mind as you eat during the day.

2. **Try to eat at least one Daily Dose (DD) of one or more of these foods each day:**

   - **Green or white tea (up to 8 cups):** Green and white tea leaves offer some of the most concentrated sources of catechins, powerful antioxidant compounds that have a proven ability to reduce body fat in men. Steeping the tea at room temperature for two hours produces a beverage that has less caffeine and bitterness and preserves catechins better than hot-brew techniques.

   - **Cinnamon (no more than 1/2 teaspoon):** Cinnamon is rich in polyphenols, which research shows have an "antidiabetic" effect. Men who consumed $\frac{1}{2}$ teaspoon of cinnamon daily for fourteen days showed improved insulin sensitivity.

   - **Oysters (up to 6):** Zinc-rich foods are linked to normal levels of testosterone and a healthy sperm count. Oysters offer the highest amount of zinc in any food; six of these tasty sea gems provide over 76 milligrams, over 500 percent of the recommended daily allowance.

   - **Cruciferous vegetables (2 handfuls):** Cruciferous vegetables like cabbage, broccoli, Brussels sprouts, kale, cress, and cauliflower contain high concentrations of glucobrassin, which turns into indole-3-carbinol (I3C), which suppresses estrogen production in men and (in animals) reduces visceral fat. Crucifers also protect your DNA and detoxify the poisons in your liver, the organ responsible for a significant number of vital functions in your body, including the production of cholesterol, from which the testes produce testosterone. Don't boil the crucifers: the indole-3-carbinol goes away. Steaming is best.

- **Hot chilies, any variety (at least I teaspoon):** Foods rich in antioxidants like red chilies, curcumin (found in the earth yellow turmeric), black pepper, cinnamon, ginger, and oregano have anti-inflammatory properties. Chilies, in particular, are full of capsaicin, a compound that promotes fat burning.

> ## MAN MEMO
> The catechins found in green tea can help prevent prostate cancer cells from forming or growing. This could be why Japanese men, who drink many cups of green tea daily, have some of the lowest rates of prostate cancer.

3. **No second portions—use only one plate per meal.** Eat from your 6-inch plate, chew your food slowly, and make eye contact with your dining partner instead of the TV. Savor your food and try not to multitask while you're eating.

> ## MAN MEMO
> Testosterone production relies a great deal on the available amounts of vitamin B and zinc in your body. Eat the right foods, and you'll ensure you're loaded for T production, without requiring supplementation. In addition to oysters, squash seeds, watermelon seeds, and pumpkin seeds are rich in zinc. For B vitamins (B_1, B_6, B_{12}, niacin, and folic acid), put these on your plate: fish, shellfish, meats, eggs, beans, and leafy green vegetables.

4. **Follow the Five Commandments (page I03).**

Phase 1 Don'ts

I. **Do not drink your calories.** No wine, beer, spirits, or other liquids with carbs or calories; this includes soda, milk, juice, and sweet teas. The only exception is your morning Classic Protein Guy Shake (page 209). There is no wiggle room here—liquid calories will crush your metabolism in a matter of sips. Just one can of Regular Coke has 39 grams of carbs—all sugar—exactly none of which has nutritional value or purpose.

Why no alcohol initially? When researchers at the University of California, San Diego, compared the habits of nearly 800 men between the ages of 50 and 9I, they found that consuming one drink or more daily lowered their testosterone levels, which stayed down for twenty-four hours. Alcohol increases the activity of testosterone reductase, a liver enzyme that breaks down testosterone. Plus, alcohol means calories without satiety. And you want satiety.

THE DISH ON DIET DRINKS

You should try to avoid most artificial sweeteners, such as those found in diet sodas. These manufactured chemicals cause appetite hormones and reward centers to respond out of turn. Go easy on sucralose (Splenda), saccharin (Sweet 'N Low), acesulfame potassium (Sunett), and aspartame (Equal, Nutra Sweet).

A good sweetener alternative but still scarce is erythritol (ZSweet), a sweet sugar alcohol: it's low in calories and doesn't give you diarrhea. If you see it, it's worth trying, as is the natural sweetener stevia. My favorite stevia brand is Trader Joe's, but Truvia and Pyure are good, too.

Honey is next best after stevia, because honey is hard to overeat, as is real maple syrup. Make sure neither is adulterated with high-fructose or other corn syrup or sweetener. Don't use the whole honey bear—try a teaspoon first before adding more.

HOT TIP

Chew xylitol-sweetened gum to clean the teeth of bacteria and help prevent cavities. Just don't let your dog blow bubbles—xylitol is toxic to canines.

INCREASING YOUR MEAL SATISFACTION

You can do anything for three days, especially something that is designed to catapult your metabolism into fat-burning mode. Your ability is there, the steps are simple (see the Refuel Easiest Steps on page 163), and your new awareness of environmental obstacles will help you create the appropriate detours. What's left? Hunger. Here's how to deal with it if it threatens your progress:

- **Pay attention to protein:** Eating enough protein is critical to feeling fuller longer. Aim to eat more fish, which promotes production of the appetite-suppressing cholecystokinin (CCK) (aka "crucial craving killer") and glucagon-like peptide-I (GLP-I). GLP-I is a hormone your body makes in the digestive tract and sends to the brain after you eat, lowering your appetite.
- **Always eat breakfast:** The importance of eating breakfast cannot be overstated. Researchers at the Harvard School of Public Health found that men who skipped

this morning meal increased by 21 percent their risk of developing type-2 diabetes. They also determined that men who ate only one or two meals a day had a greater risk than those who consumed three full meals daily. Breakfast in the morning, three square meals a day, sounds practically nostalgic, but it could be the key to setting up optimal metabolism and curbing unnecessary eating.

- **Drink more citrus or hibiscus water:** Thirst is often mistaken for hunger. If you are hungry, want a snack, or want to eat at night, go to sleep or drink more citrus water.

PHASE 1 SAMPLE MENUS

Here are a few examples of meals and snacks to eat on 2/50 days. Use these to get you started in Phase 1:

PHASE 1, SAMPLE DAY 1	
MEAL	
Breakfast	16-ounce Classic Protein Guy Shake (page 209)
	Coffee, tea, and/or citrus water
Snack (optional)	23 almonds (1 ounce)
Lunch	3 hard-cooked eggs with mustard or curry on 1 slice whole-grain bread
	1 cup cherry tomatoes
	Coffee, tea, and/or citrus water
Dinner	4 ounces grilled sirloin steak and asparagus
	Citrus water or iced or hot herbal tea

PHASE 1, SAMPLE DAY 2	
MEAL	
Breakfast	2 breakfast sausages and 2 scrambled eggs with salsa
	Coffee, tea, and/or citrus water
Snack (optional)	$\frac{1}{2}$ cup Refuel Trail Mix (see page 206)
Lunch	Sliced roasted turkey breast, spread with grainy mustard, topped with sliced almonds and rolled up in large lettuce leaves
	Apple
	Coffee, tea, and/or citrus water
Dinner	4 ounces roast chicken and 1 cup roasted Brussels sprouts
	Citrus water or iced or hot herbal tea

PHASE 1, SAMPLE DAY 3	
MEAL	
Breakfast	6 ounces smoked salmon with capers, red onion, romaine leaves, squeeze of lemon
	Coffee, tea, and/or citrus water
Snack (optional)	$\frac{1}{2}$ cup Greek yogurt topped with chopped walnuts and cinnamon
Lunch	Refuel Chicken Salad (page 221) over large bowl of mixed greens
	Coffee, tea, and/or citrus water
Dinner	$1\frac{1}{2}$ cups Central Mexican Chili (page 227)
	Citrus water or iced or hot herbal tea

RE-UP FOR PHASE 1

Apply these strategies as often as you are able. The greater your commitment, the greater your gains.

Rest

We were meant to sleep in the dark of night and wake with the light of day. If you've ever camped overnight in the near-total darkness of the wilderness, you may have experienced how natural this feels. It's part of our circadian rhythm, the sleep cycle of hormones that ties us to the natural world.

What's not natural is having nearly constant exposure to artificial light, particularly lights with a short wavelength such as those emitted by LED screens. This type of light, also referred to as blue range, creates an extended period of alertness—good when you're awake, not so good when you want to sleep. Researchers with the University of Basel in Switzerland compared LED screens to old-school non-LED ones and found that the LED screens delayed the production of melatonin and reduced sleepiness.

The problem is that we are surrounded by blue lights: flat-screen TVs, smartphone screens, and computers all emit light in this hue. Even late-night time or email checks on your smartphone can jolt you from a restful state; try to resist these habits until morning, and make a plan to stop checking at least an hour before you go to bed.

> **MAN MEMO**
>
> You'll get better sleep in front of a fire than in front of a flat-screen TV. The reddish light emitted from the flames does not affect our production of melatonin, whereas the blue light of a TV screen does.

During this phase of Refuel, make an effort to get better rest by taking these steps:

- Rid your bedroom of sources of artificial light, or at least make sure everything is powered off or camouflaged with an opaque object (e.g., a towel) before you close your eyes.
- Try to sleep in a relatively cool environment—60 to 68 degrees Fahrenheit will lower your core body temperature and help to trigger sleep.

EXERCISE

Set the stage to break a sweat tomorrow by organizing your workout gear the night before and placing it where you will see it first thing in the morning. Nothing complicated is needed clothing-wise, but an athletic-soled shoe is recommended. No tools or exercise equipment are required. To keep track of your intervals, you can simply count them to yourself or use a cellphone timer or self-tracker. Or try a cool device called GymBoss; it beeps when you need to start and when you're done, after each interval.

In this phase, you do cardio and resistance intervals on each of the three days.

PHASE I CARDIO

On each day of this phase, you walk, jog, cycle, swim, or climb for 1 minute at a warm-up pace. Then you:

- Perform 1-minute intervals for at least 5 minutes, and up to 10 minutes.
- Use a 10-second/50-second split: you go 10 seconds at 8/10 level of intensity, then 50 seconds at 2/10 level of intensity. (See p. 125 for intensity ratings.)

After your 1-minute warm-up, your 5 minutes of exercise will look like this:

PHASE 1 CARDIO INTERVALS		
MINUTE	DURATION	INTENSITY
I	10 sec.	8/10
	50 sec.	2/10
2	10 sec.	8/10
	50 sec.	2/10
3	10 sec.	8/10
	50 sec.	2/10
4	10 sec.	8/10
	50 sec.	2/10
5	10 sec.	8/10
	50 sec.	2/10

After 5 minutes, repeat once. Make certain you allow the full 50 seconds of effort at the lower level of intensity; this will allow you to push yourself hard for a total of 10 minutes.

PHASE I RESISTANCE
- Pick one of the following exercises: pushups, lunges, burpees, planks, or jumping jacks. Perform it for at least 30 seconds at 8/10 level of intensity. Rest 30 seconds, and then repeat.
- Complete 3 minutes of this resistance work each day. Your workout will look like this:

PHASE 1 RESISTANCE INTERVALS		
MINUTE	DURATION	INTENSITY
I	30 sec.	8/10
	30 sec.	Rest
2	30 sec.	8/10
	30 sec.	Rest
3	30 sec.	8/10
	30 sec.	Rest

When you're performing these resistance exercises, it's important to make them easy. If you can't do one, it's okay. Here are some modifications to get you started:

- *Pushups* should be more than a micro-bend in the elbow. If you can't achieve a 90-degree angle with your elbow, put your arms straight out and on the floor, drop to your knees, and bend your elbows to touch your chest to an imaginary fist on the floor. Do this until you can maintain proper form: back straight.
- To modify *burpees*, instead of thrusting your feet back into a pushup position, step one leg back at a time, then one at a time back to meet your hands. Stand up (don't jump) and repeat.
- To do *lunges* you can support yourself with chairs if you feel unstable. Grab two chairs (without wheels), placing one on your left and one on your right, with the chair backs facing you. Only bend at the knee until you hit 90 degrees; if all you can do is 10 degrees, that's fine—that's where you are starting. Place your hands on the top of the chairs as needed. Test the chairs' stability by applying only a little pressure at first.
- Full *jumping jacks* can be cut down to a half jack. Do this especially if you have shoulder problems. Instead of bringing your arms above your head, stop at shoulder level, palms facing down.
- *Planks* can be started as pushups that you just hold, with your arms locked. Do this especially if you have weak abdominal muscles, because leaning on your forearms and tightening your abs will make them sorer than just a pushup. If you can't get into full pushup position, just start from your knees. Once you can hold it for 10 seconds, try a full plank.

UNWIND

Before you go to sleep, grant yourself a transitional period. Let your thoughts lose their sharp edge. Trying to resolve a difficult work problem right before you attempt sleep is counterproductive. So, too, is staring at a bright screen, watching violent TV programs, or playing video games.

During Phase 1, read or watch something nonviolent and not work related for 5 minutes or more. Take three deep breaths, lying in bed flat on your back. If this prescribed idle time is too much or too uncomfortable, pick up a book, magazine, or newspaper and read a bit. Just be sure to stay away from the financial section and housing reports! Maybe the sports section, too.

PHASE 2: BOOST GROWTH HORMONE AND TESTOSTERONE (14 DAYS)

You've applied the steps of Refuel for three days, and significant metabolic shifts have already occurred. Smart and purposeful cuts in your consumption of sugar and other junky carbs have helped to regulate your insulin response, thereby putting the brakes on your fat storage. You have also been successful at shrinking your abdominal fat cells, which have slowed down the testosterone-to-estrogen conversion that was likely on high speed before.

Now, in the second phase of the plan, you will naturally boost your growth hormone and testosterone production. This happens as a metabolic response to the loss of visceral fat. Besides producing aromatase and triggering testosterone-to-estrogen conversion, that deep abdominal fat has been shown to reduce secretion of growth hormone.

Growth hormone plays a major role in many important metabolic functions. It promotes growth of muscle tissue, influences bone and cell regeneration, stimulates the oxidation of fat cells, and helps maintain stable levels of blood sugar. You need it, you want it, you got it. Without injections.

THE DANGERS OF HGH INJECTIONS

Human growth hormone (HGH) levels are highest when we are young and are still growing in height. Children who are deficient in growth hormone are treated with daily injections to boost height; a boy who is genetically set to grow to 5'3" could instead hit 5'7" if treated before puberty.

You've most likely read about athletes who have been caught using HGH injections for increased athletic performance. Or, heard about celebrities who use it to chase their fleeting youth. These aren't instances of people looking to correct a deficiency; rather, they want to supplement what they may be losing naturally through age.

The American Association of Clinical Endocrinologists published their position on this trend, stating that growth hormone was "no fountain of youth." They endorsed the use of injections only for individuals with growth hormone deficiency. And the research reveals why. Supplemental HGH has been connected to increased risk for type-2 diabetes, insulin resistance, and joint pain.

So, increase your levels of HGH naturally, with Refuel. Focus on eating well, exercising, upping your productivity, and getting quality sleep.

Italian researchers writing in the journal *Metabolism* found that high circulating levels of insulin—present when your diet is high in processed carbs—directly blunt the production of growth hormone. For this reason, the plan is for you to continue applying the 2/50 Technique (page 112) and stick with the Five Refuel Commandments (page 103) during this second phase. But that's not all. I've added simple, straightforward steps that will help push your progress forward. First, here are the dos and don'ts for this phase.

PHASE 2 DOS AND DON'TS

Phase 2 Dos

1. **Apply the 2/50 Technique for two days out of each seven days.** You've heard plenty of reasons for eating 50 grams of carbs for two days in a week, but there's more: pleasure. You enjoy carbs more when you haven't had much of them in the last two days. It's proven that the taste of something improves when you can't have it right away—the food version of absence makes the heart grow fonder. I'm not talking about forty days and forty nights; just 48 hours of monitoring your carbs, followed by five days of moderate carb consumption. Part of the pleasure comes from learning how to savor your food: you chew more, taste more, sit down to improve satiety. You'll remember your meals when they mean something to you.

2. **Take 500 mg of vitamin C and 1,000 IU of vitamin D₃ daily.** When researchers evaluated the impact of macro- and micronutrients on growth hormone, they found a significant positive association with GH secretion and vitamin C. Writing in the March 2012 issue of *Growth Hormone & IGF Research,* they noted: "vitamin C intake [is] strongly and uniquely associated with stimulated and endogenous spontaneous GH secretion." So, to enhance growth hormone production, you should take 250 milligrams of vitamin C twice daily. And as I've explained elsewhere, low vitamin D levels are associated with obesity and with lower testosterone levels. So, you take vitamin D₃ supplements that are marked with "USP" or "NSF" on the label and that come from large manufacturers. (See the Refuel Supplement Guide, starting on page 164, for additional supplement recommendations.)

3. **Snack on seeds and nuts, mini protein boosts, and a little whole fresh fruit.** Plan ahead, so you can snack on what you want to eat and not just on what you can scavenge around your office or home. A few quick and simple options are listed here, along with smarter fruit choices. Don't let the words *nonfat* and *low-fat* fool you: most products labeled as such are not much lower in calories and are often much lower in flavor. Buy regular or full-fat "bad" snack foods, if you have to have them, and eat fewer of them or throw away the bag after you've had your portion. Fresh fruit should be savored: it's high in sugar, but high in many nutrients too, and usually low in calories.

BEST SNACKS	
Pumpkin seeds	Almonds, cashews, walnuts
Squash seeds	(preferably sold in the shell)
Watermelon seeds	Citrus water
Pistachios (sold in the shell)	Hard-cooked eggs
	Cheese sticks or rounds

BEST WHOLE FRUITS	
Fresh or frozen berries (strawberries, raspberries, cranberries, blackberries, blueberries)	Fresh stone fruits (apricots, nectarines, peaches)
Fresh citrus fruits (grapefruit, lemon, lime, tangerine, clementines, kumquat)	Fresh cantaloupe, honeydew, casaba melon
	Watermelon
Apples	Avocados
	Fresh rhubarb, unsweetened

4. **Get familiar with food labels.** Food labels provide data that can make Refuel easier. Your first choices should be foods without labels indicating any processing—fresh produce and meats. When you grab any packaged food, flip it over to take a look. A rule to follow: multiply the number of servings listed in the nutritional panel by the number of calories per serving. That's the total calories in the package. Then decide how many servings the package actually looks like to you. Divide that number into the total calories, and you'll determine whether that food is worth it. A most-of-the-time rule: choose labeled options that have more protein than sugar.

   If you want to dig deeper into ingredients lists and food additives, download the free "Chemical Cuisine" app from the Center for Science in the Public Interest (CSPI). It offers an impressive amount of information and great insights, revealing what butylated hydroxytoluene and caramel coloring and other such additives really are, and giving their pros and cons.

> **HOT TIP**
> Eating a 5½-ounce serving of red meat or processed meat each day has been associated with increased risk of colon cancer. One simple way to start scaling back on your meat consumption is to try meatless Mondays, featuring tofu or another legume- or vegetable-centered dish.

5. **Follow the Commandments (page 103).**

▶ I'M SOY CONFUSED

The topic of soy and men has garnered some sensationalized stories. Soy is often called out for its "feminizing" effects, but it's more likely that environmental pollutants are to blame. In truth, first-rate human studies on soy foods are limited, but those we do have suggest that soy may help lower cholesterol, prevent cancer, increase bone density, and protect the kidneys of people with diabetes. And soy probably does not hurt thyroid function, unless you're not getting enough iodine, as is the case with many women between the ages of 20 and 39; iodized salt, seafood, and dairy can solve that problem. So, should you eat soy? My answer is yes, but with two very important caveats:

1. **Say Yes to whole, real soy.** The Okinawans (Japanese) are the world's longest-lived people, probably in part because of their diet. For millennia, they've eaten whole, organic, and fermented soy foods like miso, tempeh, tofu, and fresh edamame (young soybeans in the pod). If you consume soy foods, choose those that have been fermented and produced from non–genetically modified organisms (GMO). One to two servings (not pounds) a day of any of these foods gets the job done.

2. **Say No to processed soy.** Processed soy includes soy protein isolate and concentrates, genetically engineered soy foods (typically made from Monsanto's Roundup Ready soybeans), soy supplements, and soy food-like substances like soy cheese, soy ice cream, soy oil, and most soy burgers. If you drink soymilk, choose the unsweetened, but keep your consumption at two servings or fewer per day. These highly processed soy foods don't have the thousands of years of traditional use that whole and fermented soy foods do, and they often contain unhealthy additives and other compounds. I have real concerns about these types of soy.

Phase 2 Don'ts

1. **Don't eat hot food that comes in plastic packaging or heat food in plastic containers.** If you eat takeout hot food, don't eat it from the plastic container: transfer it to a nonplastic plate or bowl and rewarm it in a ceramic, cast-iron, or stainless-steel pot or pan. Packaged salads and never-been-hot foods are okay. Many plastics contain phthalates and BPA, known endocrine disrupters that mimic estrogen and cause chemical and metabolic confusion in your body. Scaling back your exposure to chemicals with estrogenic properties is just as important as boosting your T.

2. **Don't eat or drink while standing, lying down, walking, working at the computer, or watching TV.** Practice sitting down when you eat, no matter where you are, with your meal on a plate. If you are in front of the TV or computer or other device, move somewhere so you are not. And keep the TV turned off during dining. In one set of Cornell studies, when the TV was on, people ate 40 percent more—it was mindless eating. Tune out the tube and tune in to your food, and you'll eat less without even realizing it.

PHASE 2 SAMPLE MENUS

Here are some meal options for your second phase of Refuel: Day 1 will provide you with about 50 grams of carbohydrates; Days 2 and 3 are best to follow on the days on which you will eat 150 to 200 grams of carbs.

PHASE 2, SAMPLE DAY 1	
MEAL	
Breakfast	Breakfast quesadilla: corn tortilla, eggs, black beans, salsa, queso fresco (a mild Mexican cheese)
	Coffee, tea, and/or citrus water
Snack (optional)	Half an avocado with vinaigrette dressing
Lunch	Fish, seafood, or chicken kebabs with vegetables
	Green salad with capers, crumbled blue cheese, and red onion
	Coffee, tea, and/or citrus water
Dinner	Refuel Beef Stew (page 224)
	Citrus water or iced or hot herbal tea

PHASE 2, SAMPLE DAY 2	
MEAL	
Breakfast	Classic Protein Guy Shake (page 209)
	Coffee, tea, and/or citrus water
Snack (optional)	Cup of vegetable or lentil soup
Lunch	Stir-fried chicken with extra veggies and about $\frac{1}{2}$ cup of cooked brown or wild rice
	Citrus water or iced or hot herbal tea
Dinner	Pan-Seared Mahimahi or Halibut with Red Cabbage (page 217)
	Citrus water or iced or hot herbal tea
Dessert	Coconut Rice Pudding with Bourbon and Toasted Pecans (page 228)

PHASE 2, SAMPLE DAY 3	
MEAL	
Breakfast	Scrambled eggs and a salmon burger
	½ avocado with salsa
	Fresh mixed berries
Snack (optional)	Turkey jerky
Lunch	Scallops and mixed veggies steamed in green tea
	Miso soup
	Citrus water or iced or hot herbal tea
Dinner	Grass-fed burgers, open-faced
	Kale and parmesan salad with olive oil and lemon
	Mixed berries and walnuts with cinnamon
	Citrus water or iced or hot herbal tea

RE-UP FOR PHASE 2

Rest

Ah, sleep: it's more than a dream. Both T and GH are produced just before REM sleep. During this deep stage of sleep, GH secretion surges and T production rises. Both good.

But the less you sleep, the lower your testosterone levels. Too little sleep also increases levels of leptin and decreases levels of ghrelin, both of which will make you hungrier during the day. Fragmented sleep can disrupt your progress, so setting the stage for a solid night of sleep is key.

Counting sheep isn't the best way to sweet dreams, but there are smart steps you can take:

- Cut off the caffeine by 2:00 P.M. (and alcohol and nicotine altogether, if you are for some reason using them).
- Exercise, but do so at least 4 hours before bed.
- Avoid daytime napping.
- Don't stay in bed more than 20 minutes if you are awake and can't go back to sleep: get up and do something relaxing, like reading.

During the next fourteen days, apply this strategy to help you stick with this phase: pick two nights each week on which you can go to bed 30 minutes earlier than usual, and do so.

Exercise

Try to push the time and intensity up during this phase. Keep in mind that you don't have to stick to a set goal during the entire phase; you can start with fewer minutes and crank it up as your fitness improves. **In this phase, you do cardio and resistance intervals on twelve days of the total fourteen; you take two days off.**

PHASE 2 CARDIO

Select from one of these cardiovascular activities: walking, jogging, cycling, swimming, or climbing.

- Perform the activity for 1 minute at a warm-up pace. Then complete your cardio intervals, this time upping the cardio duration to 10 to 15 minutes total.
- Try for increased intensity as well, following a 15/45 split: 15 seconds = 8/10 level of intensity, 45 seconds = 2/10 level.

Here's how the first 5 minutes of Phase 2 Cardio would look (repeat this two or three times to hit your total time goal):

PHASE 2 CARDIO INTERVALS		
MINUTE	DURATION	INTENSITY
1	15 sec.	8/10
	45 sec.	2/10
2	15 sec.	8/10
	45 sec.	2/10
3	15 sec.	8/10
	45 sec.	2/10
4	15 sec.	8/10
	45 sec.	2/10
5	15 sec.	8/10
	45 sec.	2/10

PHASE 2 RESISTANCE

Pick two of the following exercises: pushups, lunges, burpees, planks, or jumping jacks.

- Perform the activity for at least 30 seconds at 8/10 level of intensity. Rest 30 seconds, and then do the other. Repeat.
- Increase your resistance workout duration to 4 minutes total. Here's your full workout:

PHASE 2 RESISTANCE INTERVALS		
MINUTE	DURATION	INTENSITY
1	30 sec.	8/10
	30 sec.	Rest
2	30 sec.	8/10
	30 sec.	Rest
3	30 sec.	8/10
	30 sec.	Rest
4	30 sec.	8/10
	30 sec.	Rest

Unwind

Let's build on your productivity enhancers during this phase. Continue to try to read or watch something nonviolent and not work related for five minutes or more before you go to sleep. Do one of these:

- Practice pausing before reacting to an irritating event by saying "I'm thinking about what you said/what just happened." Count to 10 to yourself as you exhale, and then respond. Work on minimizing reactions and responding instead.
- Come up with your own time-buying code word, similar to my patient's "Thank you." A simple "Right" or "Let me think" works; no need to complicate what is mostly likely an already tense moment.

With either option, the intent is the same—to move yourself into a space from which you can respond productively and capably.

10

PHASE 3: MAXIMIZE ENERGY
(7 DAYS)

Congratulations on completing the first seventeen days of Refuel. No doubt by now you've shown your belly who's boss. You've felt the snugness ease up a bit in your pants. Maybe you've even worked your way over a couple of notches on your belt. I know what those accomplishments feel like and what it takes to earn them; a tip of the hat to you for your efforts. You are upgrading your body.

Phase 3 is designed for you to stay on the path. Men who've walked this trail before you found this phase the most doable and enjoyable. They felt awakened to new habits and "life rules," as one guy put it. "The plan is becoming a lifestyle change," said another. That's the goal.

This week, you take steps to amp up your energy and improve your metabolic functions. And the roots of your Refuel program will grow deeper as you spend some skill-building time. Get ready to break out your chef's knife and steel, if you haven't already done so.

> **FAST STAT**
> Men who complete Phase 3 drop an average of l0.9 pounds over the 24 days.

PHASE 3 DOS AND DON'TS

Phase 3 Dos

1. **Apply the 2/50 Technique for two days out of seven days.** Sound familiar? You should be getting the hang of this by now: two days of 50 grams or less of carbohydrates each day, followed by five days of 150 to 200 grams each. Since you've been keeping track of your foods in a notebook or with an app, that information will be useful now.

   You've logged seven days during which you consumed only 50 grams of carbs; look back on these days and see which meals and snacks were most successful. What kept you feeling full and energized throughout the day? Which foods tasted best, and which did you truly enjoy? Which meals really worked for you? Build on those meals by replacing just one ingredient for a new taste sensation, or by adding a new spice or herb.

   Or, try something more conventional, like a pure bran cereal that is sugar free, adding berries for sweetness and toasted sliced almonds for protein. Or, mix up your routine by having something nontraditional, such as a savory meal for breakfast—more sausage patties with sage and less Day-Glo cereal. Here are a couple of my favorite options for savory breakfasts:

   - 3 chicken thighs or a salmon burger, and a cup of steamed broccoli with Sriracha
   - 2 grilled veggie burgers with a little feta, tomato, and avocado
   - 6 ounces smoked salmon, with onion, dill, capers, and horseradish

2. **Plan, choose, and eat one off-the-plan meal this week—anything you want.** This step is not meant to be an accidental indulgence. You should plan for a splurge meal so that you can anticipate looking forward to it. If you're fastidiously tracking carbs, omit this meal from your day's total tally. Say, "Sunday morning breakfast, I'm going to feast." Then savor it and celebrate—and then move on.

3. **Cook at least two dishes this week.** Whether you cook for your significant other, your kids, your parents, or just for yourself, it's time to step up to the stove. My hope is that you've found your way there already, but right now works, too.

   Pick two recipes (starting on page 209) and make them. Every guy should have a signature dish; look for two recipes that speak to you, and once you've made them both, pick one to prepare regularly and to make your own. And you don't have to stop there. Each of the recipes in this book has been crafted to provide what a man wants and needs from his food—flavor, performance, and satisfaction.

4. **Enjoy one 5-ounce glass of high-resveratrol red wine, one beer, or 1 ounce of spirits twice this week.** This is not a *must,* by any means, but wine is a wonderful thing. When paired with food, it can add richness and depth to a meal, and it will help you celebrate family, friends, and nature's gift. Red wine is rich in resveratrol, an antioxidant found in the skins of grapes, as well as in blueberries, cranberries, mulberries, lingonberries, peanuts, and pistachios. While little research has been done on humans and resveratrol, what's been published is promising:

- In the November 2011 issue of *Cell Metabolism*, researchers revealed that resveratrol supplementation (the equivalent of about 30 bottles of wine daily—not recommended) increased mitochondrial efficiency and decreased the formation of fat cells in obese men.
- A study funded by Purdue University found that piceatannol, a metabolite of resveratrol, prevented young fat cells from maturing by blocking the insulin from helping fat grow.

Even without the biochemistry, the research on wine drinking is impressive. The plant chemicals in red wine, acquired through regular, modest drinking, help prevent heart disease and slow muscle deterioration. Drink up to two glasses of wine weekly to get a head start on these benefits, or enjoy two beers or cocktails this week, but offset the calories in the alcohol by consuming 150 fewer in your food. More than two drinks weekly is not advised; excess alcohol can disrupt the quality of your sleep, lower your testosterone levels, and add calories that will become fat you feel. Sip and savor. And buy better wine; quality pays you back.

> **HOT TIP**
> The pinot noir craze has died down a bit, but this red wine should still be near the top of your list if you drink wine; it often has twice as much resveratrol as most other red wines.

5. **Find more pleasure in quality food.** Every bit of food you put in your body has a story, and that story inevitably transfers itself to your cells, tissues, and organs. Whether vegetables have been grown en masse in mineral-depleted soil or by

hand in your own backyard or window box makes a difference in how valuable the food is to your body. Whether animals have been raised humanely or not, and pumped full of antibiotics as "growth promoters," is important, too. The quality of production directly translates to the quality of the food you eat. Minimizing your exposure to toxins, drugs, and pesticides will not only improve your metabolism and decrease your levels of estrogen. It will also vastly improve your experiences with food—and this will often be immediately clear from the very first bite.

To boost the quality of food you eat, look to farmers' markets for the best fresh, seasonal produce in your area. Purchase fish, poultry, eggs, and meats that have been sustainably raised, free range, hormone free, and grass fed when possible. For example, grass-fed beef contains less overall fat than conventional, which is where the chemical pollutants get stored. Buying organic all the time can get costly, so use the Environmental Working Group's (EWG) Shopper's Guide to Pesticides in Produce (see sidebar below) to see when it's most important. If you buy nonorganic goods, try to purchase them from someone local, and then wash, wash, wash for food safety; peel off the outer skins, when appropriate.

▶ HOT TIP

Get the scoop on farmers' markets in your area at http://search.ams.usda.gov/farmersmarkets/. You'll find location, schedule, and methods of payment accepted (varies, based on information provided by each market).

▶ ENVIRONMENTAL WORKING GROUP'S SHOPPER'S GUIDE TO PESTICIDES IN PRODUCE

DIRTY DOZEN PLUS

Buy these organic:

1. Apples	8. Nectarines
2. Bell peppers	9. Peaches
3. Blueberries	10. Potatoes
4. Celery	11. Spinach
5. Cucumbers	12. Strawberries
6. Grapes	13. Green beans
7. Lettuce	14. Kale/collard greens

CLEAN FIFTEEN

Lowest in pesticides; OK to buy conventional

1. Asparagus	9. Mangoes
2. Avocados	10. Mushrooms
3. Cabbage	11. Onions
4. Cantaloupes	12. Pineapples
5. Corn	13. Sweet peas
6. Eggplant	14. Sweet potatoes
7. Grapefruit	15. Watermelons
8. Kiwi	

Source: Environmental Working Group

Phase 3 Don't

1. **Don't stop what you're doing—it's working.** For these seven days of Phase 3, it's all about the *doing*. Stay grounded to the Five Refuel Commandments (see page 103).

PHASE 3 SAMPLE MENUS

Here are some sample menus for Phase 3: Day 1 will provide you with about 50 grams of carbohydrates; Days 2 and 3 are best to follow on the days on which you will eat 150 to 200 grams of carbs.

PHASE 3, SAMPLE DAY 1

MEAL	
Breakfast	Open-faced breakfast sandwich of breakfast sausage, scrambled eggs, and grated Romano cheese on a whole wheat sandwich thin
	Coffee, tea, and/or citrus water
Snack (optional)	Roasted pumpkin seeds
Lunch	Jamaican Two-Bean Veggie Soup (page 215)
Dinner	Grilled salmon steaks with green beans topped with toasted almonds
	Citrus water or iced or hot herbal tea

PHASE 3, SAMPLE DAY 2	
MEAL	
Breakfast	Two breakfast tacos: low-carb tortilla with roasted chicken, bell pepper strips, lettuce, and Dijon mustard
	Coffee, tea, and/or citrus water
Snack (optional)	Cottage cheese with fresh fruit or tomatoes
Lunch	Two open-faced grilled veggie (or bison) burgers on romaine, with ketchup or Sriracha and sliced or cubed jicama
	Two mozzarella cheese sticks or Mini Babybel wheels
	Coffee, tea, and/or citrus water
Dinner	Grilled Sirloin Steak and Asparagus (page 222)
	Cauliflower Popcorn (page 214)
	Citrus water or iced or hot herbal tea
	Optional: 1 glass Pinot Noir

RE-UP FOR PHASE 3

Rest

Science has left little room for doubt when it comes to the connection between sleep and weight gain, which is why I want you to continue to work at developing better sleep habits. During this phase, you put all the steps together, and step it up:

- Make an effort to sleep in a dark room.
- Go to bed 30 minutes earlier two nights during this week.
- **BONUS:** Pay attention to your sleep schedule and keep it as routine as possible. Your body will respond to consistent sleep, with regular wake times and sleep triggers. For example, if you get in the habit of reading a book in bed, that will signal your body to prep for sleep.

Exercise

When researchers at the University of Georgia analyzed seventy controlled studies on exercise, 90 percent of them demonstrated a clear link between regular exercise and reduced fatigue. Indeed, exercise proved to be a consistent fatigue-fighter: in 6,800 subjects, exercise was stronger even than the stimulants used to treat ADHD and narcolepsy.

So, skip the energy drinks and get your exercise instead.

During this phase, consider your workout choices and vary them or increase the challenge when possible. If you've been jogging, increase your speed to a run for a few seconds. If you've spent most of the time doing pushups and lunges, switch to burpees and jumping jacks this week. If you raise the bar, you will continue to see improvement.

That's one of my secrets, by the way. I ask my patients, "What's your next goal?" Setting small, regular, incremental challenges—whether it's ratcheting up to an 8 in intensity today in contrast to yesterday's 7, or reaching 12,000 steps on a pedometer today instead of yesterday's 11,678, or not eating after 8:30 P.M. tonight instead of 9:00 P.M.—can help you reach beyond what you thought possible.

In this phase, you do cardio and resistance intervals on six days of the total seven; you take one day off.

> ## HOT TIP
> You don't have to use a clip-on pedometer to keep track of your steps. Many tools that track steps are now sleek and discreet. One option, called the Fitbit One, has mini measurements—just 2 inches high and ¾ inch wide. It fits in the watch pocket of your jeans (it's what that tiny pocket on your hip was designed for), and syncs with your computer and the cloud. See more tracking tools on page 131.

- Perform your chosen activity for 1 minute at a warm-up pace. Then complete your cardio intervals, maintaining the same 15/45 split intensity.
- Increase your cardio duration to 15 to 20 minutes total.

Here's how the first 5 minutes of Phase 3 Cardio would look (repeat this three or four times to hit your total time goal):

PHASE 3 CARDIO INTERVALS		
MINUTE	DURATION	INTENSITY
1	15 sec.	8/10
	45 sec.	2/10
2	15 sec.	8/10
	45 sec.	2/10

PHASE 3 CARDIO INTERVALS (continued)		
MINUTE	DURATION	INTENSITY
3	15 sec.	8/10
	45 sec.	2/10
4	15 sec.	8/10
	45 sec.	2/10
5	15 sec.	8/10
	45 sec.	2/10

PHASE 3 RESISTANCE

Pick two of the following exercises: pushups, lunges, burpees, planks, or jumping jacks.

- Perform one activity for at least 30 seconds at 8/10 level of intensity. Rest 30 seconds. Perform the other. Then repeat.
- Increase your resistance duration to 5 minutes total. Here's your full workout:

PHASE 3 RESISTANCE INTERVALS		
MINUTE	DURATION	INTENSITY
1	30 sec.	8/10
	30 sec.	Rest
2	30 sec.	8/10
	30 sec.	Rest
3	30 sec.	8/10
	30 sec.	Rest
4	30 sec.	8/10
	30 sec.	Rest
5	30 sec.	8/10
	30 sec.	Rest

Unwind

Getting better at unwinding, or better responding to stress (not getting wound up in the first place), and increasing your productivity are not about isolated successes. They are about creating a plan to make the healthiest choices also the easiest ones. That means that there's no quick fix. But if you return to the Easiest Steps (page 163) and the strategies I've outlined in Phase 1 and Phase 2, and practice them until they become default, unwinding will become easy.

During this phase, stick with what works and build upon it:

- Read or watch something nonviolent and not work-related for 5 minutes before bed. The 5-minute period is the starting point, and your goal should be to gradually add to it until your pre-sleep ritual is 30 minutes long.
- Try the *4-7-8 Belly Breath* (also described on page 61). It doesn't sound like much, but this is truly an instant shot of calm. My colleague Dr. Andrew Weil taught me this years ago, and I've taught it to many patients since; it's a way to regain balance, resolve insomnia, or rectify road rage. When you feel acutely stressed, do the following to break the tension in your muscles and rechannel the energy:

1. Inhale through your nose for 4 counts.
2. Hold your breath for a count of 7.
3. Exhale through your mouth for 8 counts.

Do this four times, up to twice daily, or as often as needed. Lengthen the time interval between each count as you get good at this: build up to at least 5 seconds.

START SMALL, BUILD BIG

Now that you know how the three phases of the 24-Day Plan work, you can jump right in with Phase 1 as soon as you take the SAM Quizzes (page 71). You can also use the quick reference guide on page 163, which lists the Refuel Easiest Steps for each phase: one step each for eating, resting, exercising, and unwinding. Apply these starter steps to form the foundation for developing new habits, and to strengthen and build on those habits as you go.

REFUEL EASIEST STEPS
PHASE 1—3 DAYS

- Eat breakfast with eggs.
- Before you brush your teeth at night, put away your phone and tablet, out of sight, until morning.
- Do 3 pushups right after you get out of bed. Do 3 more any time you feel like it.
- Take 1 chest-filling deep breath before you walk out the door for the day.

PHASE 2—14 DAYS

- Read one food label's ingredients before eating a packaged food.
- After dinner, set the alarm for 30 minutes before bedtime.
- Place your athletic gear in front of the door *or* drive to the gym rather than home after work *or* put on your running shoes in the morning first thing when you get out of bed.
- After you brush your teeth at night, put an easy-reading book on your pillow, opened to the page you want to start reading and facedown so it stays open.

PHASE 3—7 DAYS

- Right after you get up on day 18, plan your splurge meal date and time (celebration is important).
- Sleep in a dark room; after you turn off the light at night, hold your hand out in front of you—it should not be glowing.
- Go outside or into the garage or other space to do 1 minute of exercise at the end of the day, if you have not done any earlier.
- Before going into a meeting or having a potentially difficult conversation, go to the bathroom, close the stall door, and try one 4-7-8 Belly Breath.

BEFORE WE GET COOKING

Refuel is not simply about eating to lose your gut; it's about eating to discover real foods as the complete package of incredible flavors, unmatched nutrition, and deep pleasure. You'll learn how to prepare real foods with a skill that will last you a lifetime: cooking.

In Part Four of *Refuel*, we get to cooking and food. But first check out Chapter 11 on how to maximize your health by choosing the right supplements.

11

THE REFUEL SUPPLEMENT GUIDE

When it comes to dietary supplements, it's a crazy world out there—partly because supplements are not subject to the same regulations as are drugs—or even food. Almost any claims can be made. Take this pill and burn fat! Take this pill and live longer! Take this pill and your dog will stop having accidents on the rug!

Take, for example, a product called Exotica that claims to help "male sexual enhancement" by way of its secret ingredient, horny goat weed. Should you doubt the effectiveness of such a clearly potent product (the name says it all!), Exotica has the estimable endorsement of the Institute of Sexology, in France. The bonus is that you can order 500 bottles or more at a time. Should you take it? Only if you don't mind wasting money. And if you feel okay about having something called Exotica in your medicine cabinet. Needless to say, there are better investments you can make when it comes to supplements.

This chapter describes how to create and maintain a healthy vitamin and mineral balance; identifies which specific vitamins, minerals, and dietary supplements you should take; and suggests which supplements you can avoid—because they only make expensive pee and sometimes hurt your liver, nerves, or kidneys. Visit www.drjohnlapuma

.com for a printable version of the Refuel supplement guide and to find my newsletter offering additional tips and tools.

THE NEED FOR MULTIVITAMINS

Do you really need one? The short answer is yes. Get the one with no more than 100 percent of the daily value of everything in it; it should have no iron, no calcium, less than 2,500 IU of beta-carotene, and a maximum of 55 mcg of selenium (the amount found in half of one Brazil nut). Too much selenium may cause diabetes; just enough will reduce prostate cancer risk. Add extra vitamins C and D and omega-3s (see pages 167–168), and you're good to go. If you are diabetic or pre-diabetic, consider adding 1,800 mg of alpha-lipoic acid.

Supplementing is essential today because the standard American diet, while calorie rich, is quite nutrient poor. The average annual individual consumption of sweeteners is 141 pounds; pizza, 24 pounds; ice cream, 23 pounds. Sure, you might get a little calcium and protein from the cheese and ice cream, but even that's stretching it a bit. If the average person were to eat 141 pounds of spinach a year instead of sugar, our national health statistics would look nothing like they do today.

Sadly, food quality, including that of fresh produce, isn't what it used to be. Even those of us who make an effort to consume fresh fruits and vegetables are not reaping the same nutritional benefits as generations past did. The reason? Modern conventional agricultural methods deplete the soil of minerals, which translates to nutrient-depleted produce. Some hybrid varieties of plants have been modified to improve transportability, at a loss of flavor and nutrition. Nutrients are also lost as produce is shipped from farms to grocery stores, during the cooking process, and even by being exposed to air and light.

HOW TO BUY THE RIGHT MULTIVITAMINS

Before you go to the store, check your cupboard and evaluate what you already have. Check the expiration dates. Throw away any expired multivitamins.

At the store, avoid vitamins and supplements for which there is "emerging science" and that you've never heard of. Vitamin O, for example, is simply oxygen: freely available in the atmosphere or in a capsule. It's your choice.

Look for the USP or NSF symbol on the label; it's a marker of quality. Then, look for an expiration date: if it is not there, or if it has passed, put it back on the shelf or deliver it to store personnel.

Choose a multivitamin that is manufactured or distributed by a large company—a company that has a lot to lose if its quality slips. Buy a major brand or store brand. (When Consumers Union tested some cut-rate products, it found that almost half of them didn't contain the listed amounts of at least one nutrient.) Avoid "timed-released" vitamins and "chelated" minerals, which have no known clinical impact on absorption.

Look also for the serving size; if the portion size is too many capsules or tablets for you to take easily, or they need to be taken more than twice daily, put it back. Less is more; the simpler the ingredients list, the better. If you have trouble swallowing multivitamins, consider a liquid multivitamin, or chewable ones; they are often just as effective.

HOW TO TAKE YOUR MULTIVITAMINS

Once you're taking your vitamins, if you forget to take them one day, don't take a double dose to make up for it. Just go back on the schedule the next day.

Put your multivitamins in a place where it is easy for you to take them, every day—by your toothbrush, by the coffeemaker, in your desk drawer. A cool and dry place is better than a hot and humid one, if you can find it. Put the multivitamins out of reach of kids, too.

WHAT SHOULD BE IN YOUR MULTIVITAMINS

The following are the maximum intake amounts for vitamins, minerals, and fatty acids; lower amounts will also be safe. (IU is the abbreviation for International Units; mcg is the abbreviation for micrograms; mg is the abbreviation for milligrams.) Note: after age 50, men and women can take the same multivitamin.

Vitamins

- A: No more than 2,500 IU (1.6 mg) daily. Men who ingest an average of more than 4,300 IU daily have a dramatically increased risk of hip fracture over those who ingest the least. Too much vitamin A also increases the risk for lung and liver cancers. If you smoke, it also increases your risk for stroke. This is true for supplements, but not for food.
- B_6: No more than 2 mg daily.
- B_{12}: No more than 25 mcg daily in a supplement. (B_{12} in a supplement is absorbed much better than the B_{12} found in food; it is not toxic.)
- C: Approximately 250 mg twice daily.
- D: 1000 IU daily, vitamin D_3 preferred. (Unless you have kidney stones, and then less than 200 IU daily.) Men with vitamin D deficiency have lower total T and higher estrogen levels; get your D checked. Ask your doctor for a 25-hydroxy vitamin D blood test, or get one online (several options are available at www.drjohnlapuma.com); make sure you get a blood test.
- E: No more than 60 IU twice daily, mixed tocopherols preferred. (Skip if you are taking a statin drug.) Don't take more than this: over 400 IU boosts risk for prostate cancer.
- F (folate or vitamin B_9): 400 mcg daily.

> **HOT TIP**
> Snack on sunflower seeds to get natural vitamin E. Just $\frac{1}{4}$ cup provides nearly 100 percent of the recommended daily allowance.

Minerals

- Calcium: Tread cautiously: limit your calcium from supplements to lower the risk of kidney stones and aggressive prostate cancer. (Calcium from food does not increase risk of kidney stones and may lower it.) On the other hand, men with low calcium intake are more likely to gain weight, have a higher body mass index, and be overweight or obese compared to people with higher calcium intake. Aim for no more than 500 to 600 mg daily, and feel good about getting it from food instead of as a supplement; try added-sugar-free Greek yogurt, almond milk, leafy greens.
- Magnesium: 400 mg daily (although this is better obtained from food, especially nuts and seeds).

- Selenium: Up to 55 mcg daily (but none if you have had invasive squamous cell skin cancer).
- Zinc: 11 mg daily. (Too much zinc, however, suppresses immunity, so don't overdo it.)

> ### MAN MEMO
> Too much heme iron in your body is far worse than too little: it increases the risk for diabetes. Approximately two 4-ounce servings of red meat weekly will supply you with enough iron.

Essential Fatty Acids

Omega-3s: up to 2 g of fish oil total daily, with at least 600 mg of DHA, which is the most powerful component of fish oil; vegetarians can get it from algal oil. (Those on anticoagulants such as warfarin, or who take flax, fish, black currant, borage, or evening primrose oil, should have their coagulation status monitored by their physician.)

Omega-3s can lower triglyceride levels so well that there are prescription medications made from them for this purpose—ask your doctor about this option if you have high triglycerides.

WHAT SHOULD NOT BE IN YOUR MULTIVITAMIN

- Any Iron: An oxidant and it increases damage to your blood vessels; in men, it increases the risk of gallstones.
- Any Copper: Linked more than any mineral in studies of multivitamins to an increased risk of death.
- More than 2,500 IU Beta-Carotene daily: Two large studies have found that supplemental beta-carotene increased lung cancer, and increased risk of death in people who smoked and in men who worked with asbestos.
- More than 100 mg of Vitamin B_6 daily: Peripheral neuropathy (pain and numbness in extremities) is a common side effect; fortunately, that often goes away when the vitamin is discontinued.
- More than 40 mg of Zinc: This is the upper limit; too much interferes with absorption and does not help testosterone production.

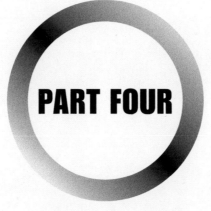

PART FOUR

GET REAL

THE SIMPLE PATH TO ENJOYING THE FOOD YOU LOVE

COOKING IS FREEDOM

Five Easy Cooking Techniques and the Tools You'll Need to Man a Kitchen

I have the yen for cooking and eating in my genes. My grandfather, his father, and his father were all bakers. My dad used to make homemade yogurt in an oven warmed by its pilot for my five siblings and me when we were kids; my mom would pressure-cook dried soybeans and pull fresh greens (aka weeds) for salads from the garden. Meals were cooked and eaten at home, out of both ritual and necessity—we couldn't afford to eat out. We saw fruits and vegetables as staples, and we learned to view the tops of turnips, the peels of pumpkins, and the onion skins not as trash but as precious ingredients in our compost piles and then in a new crop.

The message was this: we have the instinct and the skills to take care of ourselves. As a third-generation Italian American, I saw this partly as a product of adaptation, carried over from a time when taking charge of one's survival wasn't optional. So I did take care of myself, and by the time I was in my thirties, I had worked hard enough to establish a promising career in medical ethics. Yet, I was leading an unbalanced life. My belly was growing and my energy and sex drive were diminishing. Not being able to manage my own weight, I felt better referring my overweight and obese patients to dietitians instead of treating them myself. I was at a crossroads.

BACK TO THE CUTTING BOARD

I realized that the skill missing in my life was the one that was most personal to me: cooking. I needed to break out of my routine and chop, crush, sauté, season, and macerate, even though I hardly knew what those terms were. So I went back to school to study as a chef.

Learning how to cook brought me back to the pleasures I'd neglected, renewed my confidence, and gave me profound satisfaction. Cooking proved to be just as complex and interesting as medicine, requiring the same attentiveness and care. No matter how small the job, with cooking you always have something to show for your efforts. And the disappointments, which are inevitable, can be tossed if need be, and chalked up to the learning curve.

The more I cooked, the deeper grew my appreciation for unprocessed foods and the better my pants fit. The correlation goes beyond my own experience. Cooking is satisfying because it offers a sense of control and confidence. And the fastest route to improved eating is by way of cooking. Sure, there are shortcuts, but most shortcuts aren't anchored to skill development or expertise.

I'm not suggesting you have to cook every day or all the time (unless you want to). But being able to cook a few staples should be in your arsenal. A man who can cook is a self-sufficient, capable provider, which is about as masculine as it gets. Just ask Bobby Flay, Emeril Lagasse, Wolfgang Puck, Anthony Bourdain, Mario Batali, or Gordon Ramsay. These guys come to life when they are surrounded by sharp steel knives and fire-hot grills, and they get their culinary thrills by balancing flavors and creating something amazing in seemingly impossible circumstances. You can, too. To get started, I'm going to teach you the most essential skills with minimal fuss that will give you the foundation you need.

Before you step right into the fire, however, you've got to outfit your kitchen with the essential and most useful tools. As with other types of tools—whether they're for sports or for fixing up things around the house—you'll discover that there are those you need and others you just *want*. (There is such a thing as chef's knife envy.)

HOW TO "MAN" YOUR KITCHEN—THE BARE ESSENTIALS

Start by taking a kitchen inventory to find out what you do and do not need. Grab an empty box and be prepared to lighten the load in the cooking zone. A word of warning: it's best to consult your significant other before delivering half the kitchen's contents to the local Goodwill.

There are undoubtedly items in your kitchen that have never been used, or should no longer be used. That fondue set you got years ago as a wedding or anniversary gift? Donate it. The chipped beer mug from college? Time to let it go. Half a box of plastic forks left over from a picnic? Gone. Rusty colander or grater? Toss 'em. Aim for fewer items of better quality. Apply the same scrutiny to your cabinets.

Check your nonstick pots and pans for scratches. Any with severe gashes, gaps, or other damage should be disposed of. At high heat, nonstick pans release toxic gases; these are even more likely to be released if the pan is damaged. Plus, bits of the nonstick coating can break off into your food—not good for flavor or texture, much less your immune system.

You can get by without applying this swift scan-and-scrap step, but creating a clutter-free culinary workshop is worth the time it takes. Ever searched in a hurry for a pen in a messy drawer? Imagine that magnified exponentially as you watch the ribeyes burn while you search for the tongs.

Now, let's get to the essential tools needed for your kitchen. Items are listed in order of priority. Buy what you can and build from there. See more of my ideas for your kitchen, including brand recommendations, online.

Here are the bare essentials.

1. Chef's knife and honing steel
2. Blender
3. Tongs
4. Heavy-bottomed 6-quart Dutch oven

With these four tools (the knife and steel are paired, as you'll see), you can make a lifetime of meals—and more than a few memorable ones. The great thing about home-cooked meals is that they almost always taste good—sure, they can be *not great*, but bad is rare. Bad only happens when the top pops off of the oregano jar and the entire contents spill into your spaghetti sauce; or instead of adding chili powder, you pour on the cinnamon. But adventures in cooking beget adventures in eating. Maybe a kick of cinnamon will go really nicely with a spicy carne asada (marinated grilled meat). An open mind will serve you well as you step up to the stove (and the plate).

▶ SAFETY IN THE KITCHEN

I sometimes ask audiences: What's the most important safety tool to have in the kitchen? You'd be surprised how many people don't know the answer. Knife slipups and cuts can be awful, but the risk of fire is the most dangerous possibility in the kitchen. If you don't already have one within quick reach in the kitchen, get a fire extinguisher. Do it today.

Chef's Knife and Honing Steel

These two go together like Muhammad Ali and Angelo Dundee. A good chef's knife will slice and dice ingredients with swift skill. There is one caveat: you have to know how to use it. A honing steel will whip the blade back into shape in a matter of minutes. Buy wisely here because these two tools won't be sitting long between rounds; in fact, they're just waiting for the bell. Here's what to look for in each.

Chef's knives come in two varieties: forged and stamped. A *forged* knife has been hammered or forged from one piece of metal, which makes it feel solid. A forged knife will typically, though not always, have a bolster or metal lip that curls up at the top of the handle. *Stamped* knives are produced from one large continuous sheet of steel, which is "stamped" by a machine to create the blades (imagine a knife-shaped cookie cutter). A forged blade is generally stronger and heavier, with no flexibility. A stamped knife will be lighter and have some flexibility. Stamped knives can be easier to use with speed and are less expensive.

So, which is better? You'll find passionate camps in both corners of the ring, but I say it all comes down to personal preference. A chef's knife should be thought of as an extension of your hand, so it's most important to choose what feels best to you.

To pick the piece that best suits you, duck into a Macy's, T.J. Maxx, or Sears and give a few knives a trial grip. You want the knife short enough to maneuver with confidence ("it's not size, but what you can do with it" applies here as well). Take hold of a 7- or 8-inch chef's knife. Grip the handle like you're shaking someone's hand—this is the grip that will give you the most control—and see how the weight and balance feel.

My favorite knife is made by Victorinox Forschner; they have durable, high-quality stamped lightweight knives for less than $50. Other great brands are J.A. Henckels, Wüsthof, and Cuisinart. Wherever your brand preference guides you, get a blade that's made of high-carbon stainless steel, as others rust and get dull quicker.

Where to keep your knife? In a wooden block or a BladeSafe, a type of knife sheath made from rugged polypropylene. For the latter, put one of these on your blade before storing it in a drawer—it's better for the blade and you'll eliminate the risk of unpleasant nicks and cuts as you search for a spatula.

THE RIGHT WAY TO USE A KNIFE

You've sliced plenty of sandwiches in half, and maybe carved a turkey, but getting a recap on the basics never hurt anyone. Here's how to practice your knife skills. (You can also check out www.drjohnlapuma.com to watch demonstrations of those skills.)

1. Place a damp towel under a cutting board (to prevent slippage) and set a celery stick on the surface, lengthwise in front of you, flat side down.
2. Grip the knife handle with your dominant hand and place the opposite hand on the celery.
3. Bend your opposite hand's fingers until they resemble a half-fist. Keep your fingertips tucked the entire time you're cutting.
4. Place the tip of the knife on the board behind the celery, and nudge the blade right up against the knuckles of your tucked hand.

5. Begin cutting with a fluid rocking (no sawing or hacking) motion, stabilizing the celery with your noncutting hand as you move down the line.

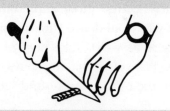

Knife time: put both hands to work and you'll be a more efficient cutting machine.

Keep in mind that you want to anchor the cutting motion in your shoulder and back, not your arm and wrist—think more of a long tennis swing than a quick baseball cut. While speed slicing and dicing has its allure, a tipless finger is not so appealing—start slowly and speed will come with practice.

To maintain your knife's form, get a honing steel. The most important factor here is the strength of the steel—the honing steel must be harder than the knife for it to work. This is why I recommend getting the knife and steel as a paired set, or at least from the same manufacturer.

Different from sharpening, honing splits off unwanted microscopic burrs from the edge of a blade, giving you a consistently cleaner cut. You should hone the blade's edge every time you use your chef's knife.

To hone a knife blade's edge:

1. Point the honing steel away from your body so that it's perpendicular to your torso.
2. Hold the knife blade at about a 20-degree angle to the steel.
3. Place the heel of the knife at the base of the steel, near its handle, with the blade facing away from you (others instructions will recommend you hold it toward the body, but away is much safer until you get the hang of the motion).
4. Move one side of the blade with light pressure on the edge up the steel moving away from you. Finish so that the tip of the knife ends near the tip of the steel.

5. Repeat two to five times.
6. Switch to the other side of the blade. Repeat two to five times.
7. Clean the steel with a dish towel after each use; if you don't do this, the filings will build up and diminish the knife's effectiveness, and even damage the blade. Watch a quick clip of how to hone a knife at www .drjohnlapuma.com.

First rule of knife club: keep the blade facing away from your body.

A knife sharpening, on the other hand, should be done only once a year because it wears down the metal to renew the "V" of the blade edge. Get this sharpening done by a professional, since an overzealous sharpening job can take years off the life of your knife. Plus, professional sharpening services are inexpensive—an 8-inch knife will typically cost between $4 and $8.

THE SHARPEST TOOL IS THE SAFEST

Don't let a dull blade happen to you. A dull knife is probably the leading cause of accidents in the kitchen (next to small children or animals running around, and maybe tequila drinking). Here's why sharpest is safest:

- You will have inherently greater respect for a sharp knife. A sharp blade commands attention and awareness, two factors that will make you a safer, smarter, and better cook.
- A sharp knife cuts cleaner. Instead of tearing flesh, cells, and tissues, it slices through them, leading to less slipping and chance of injury. And you'll have fewer tears when dicing onions.

> **CHEF'S SECRET**

Here's the protocol for care of your chef's knife: hone, use, wash, wipe, store.

Hone, we've covered (page 176). Use, ditto (page 175). To wash, apply a quick rinse after you're done slicing and dicing. Wipe with a soft towel, but try not to wipe the edge; it hurts—you and the blade. Wipe away from you, starting at the bolster and moving toward the point. Then, to store the knife, put it in a knife block, in a drawer with knife separator partitions, or on a magnetic bar.

Three other rules for using a knife:

1. Don't wash it in the dishwasher: it cracks the handle and dulls the blade.
2. Don't store it haphazardly in a kitchen drawer. It is dangerous and may nick the blade.
3. Don't bring a knife to a gunfight. (Also, don't go to gunfights at all.)

Blender

The blender is one of the most versatile tools to have in your kitchen. You can use this awesome machine to puree vegetables for soups, make quick and simple salsas and salad dressings, chop vegetables if you're tight on time (although a food processor is better for this if you have one), and blend meal-equivalent shakes and smoothies. The Classic Protein Guy Shake (page 209) is so good, it's sure to whip any blender into shape. Here are a few things to look for:

- **A removable blade.** Instead of digging around under the blades with your fingers to remove trapped food, look for blades that pop out for cleaning if you're using an ordinary blender (as opposed to a turbocharged one).
- **An hourglass figure.** Or half of one—the best blenders taper down so all the ingredients are funneled in evenly.
- **A racing pulse.** This super-speed button allows you to add the finishing touches on a shake without ending up with a fruit-flavored puddle.
- **A propeller blade.** This blade allows foods to drop down into the blades. The other common design is the "star" blade, which can actually trap ingredients and prevent them from getting processed. If you get this type of blender, make sure it comes with a tamper to use through the top.

- **A top with a removable center.** The removable center piece is often a measuring device, and can be removed to allow you to pour in ingredients while you are blending. It must be removed before you blend hot liquids. (I like to cover the opening firmly with a towel before blending hot liquids.)

I especially like blenders made by Braun, KitchenAid, and Breville. And if you want to go for the cream of the crop, get a Vitamix. It's easy to clean and can be used as juicer to boot. The Vitamix is an investment, costing close to $500, but the seven-year warranty gives you some time to work out any mechanical kinks without incurring additional cost.

> **CHEF'S SECRET**
> Look for a blender that comes with a glass or BPA-free container. As I like to say,
> "No estrogen in my shake, thanks."

Tongs

The ultimate functional hand tool, tongs have many uses beyond the quick flip of a steak or chicken breast. You can use tongs to mix, toss, scramble, push, nudge, sample, and sauté (but keep metal-tipped ones off of nonstick pans). Buy multiple pairs, if you can. This way, you'll have a backup when one is in the dishwasher or left hanging outside on the barbecue. Wooden and metal tongs work extremely well; I avoid plastic ones for the chemical uncertainty, but silicone are okay as long as they have a nontoxic coating. If you only get one pair, grab the shorter version. A short pair of super sturdy stainless-steel tongs will provide more versatility and be easier to maneuver than the huge but unwieldy aluminum/wood/leather/giant tongs so commonly on sale in early June.

Locking tongs store more easily in drawers, but I have multiple pairs of tongs resting in a ceramic utensil holder by the stove. The ones I reach for most are the 9-inchers made by Oxo and All-Clad.

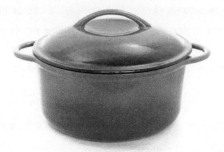

A sturdy Dutch oven will outlast half a dozen electric razors.

Heavy-Bottomed 6-Quart Dutch Oven

If you can have only one pot in your kitchen, it should be a 6-quart Dutch oven. Literally a mini-oven, this workhorse piece of cookware has been around for hundreds of years. It has been an essential traveling companion for men of adventure, helping feed Lewis and Clark and their team, and countless mountaineers and cowboys.

What's so great about this pot? Well, it can be used for boiling, stewing, roasting, baking, sautéing, simmering, and braising. You can marinate meats in most Dutch ovens since they don't absorb flavor or odors if they are lined with ceramic or are pure stainless steel. After cooking, you can serve meals straight from the pot. Want to preserve the leftovers of a one-pot meal? You should. Cover, place in the refrigerator after it cools, and then the next day, just slide it right back onto the stove for reheating. If you get the enameled cast-iron Dutch oven, you've also picked up the perfect tool for cooking practice—it cleans very easily. Skip the nonstick versions: you don't need the toxic fumes.

You should think of the purchase of a Dutch oven as an investment. A high-quality heavy-duty one by a well-known brand, like the ceramic-lined Le Creuset, will run upwards of $150, but this is a piece you can pass on to your children. I love the All-Clad stainless-steel version: it doubles as a boiling or simmering pot, which would take a lot longer in a cast-iron anything. Plus the All-Clad is light and just 5.5 quarts, a good size. But it, too, is expensive.

You can also find less expensive, well-reviewed Dutch ovens for around $60. Consider Lodge for the pure cast-iron and Tramontina for the enamel-lined cast iron; they're big, brawny, and beautiful. Just be sure to check the surface for chips on the enameled variety, as there have been reports of missing coating on less expensive varieties.

CHEF'S SECRET

Most Refuel staple cookware is durable and designed to last years. However, one careless mistake can ruin a treated pot or pan for good. Pretend it's 1965 and read the manual, making careful note of the instructions for use and cleaning. You'll get more out of your investment this way.

THE SECOND STRING

When you've compiled your essentials, add to your kitchen from this list of nice-to-haves, which may eventually become essential goods:

- **Wooden spoons:** these are great for stirring and sautéing, plus they won't scratch pots.
- **Two cutting boards:** a BPA-free (look at product labeling) plastic cutting board for meat, fish, shellfish, and poultry; a wood one for everything else.
- **Serrated knife:** the best for bread and slicing through tomato skin.
- **Medium saucepan:** pony up for 18/8 or 18/10 (they're basically the same) stainless steel. Copper is not worth the extra cost or cleaning hassle.
- **Stainless-steel skillet:** a skillet has flared out edges, different from a saucepan, which has straight edges. The skillet is lighter, but has less cooking surface. If you can, get both. A skillet is best for browning.
- **Box grater:** a box grater is sturdier than a microplane and is great for grating sweet potatoes and zesting citrus.
- **Meat thermometer:** when you want your meat medium rare, well done can be dryly disappointing.
- **Colander:** you could drain out water using the pan lid, but why should you if you don't have to? Look for rust-free stainless steel or colanders made from BPA-free plastic, such as those from Preserve or Endurance.
- **Mixing bowls:** stainless steel is best—indestructible. These are great for making dressings, sauces, and salads, and for tossing vegetables with seasonings pre-roasting.
- **Jelly roll pan/baking sheet:** a thicker version of the cookie sheet with higher edges, perfect for roasting or warming frozen hors d'oeuvres.

Start with the essentials, and then add as your budget allows (see sidebar, page 183) and skill demands. Cooking is like a sport—tools of the trade will get you only so far without skill. You could put a $300 glove made from the finest kangaroo leather on an unskilled guy, and Derek Jeter and a sock would still out-field him. Let's get to the fundamental five cooking techniques.

> **ON MAN DUTY**
> If you're taking on more responsibilities around the house these days, you're not alone. More families are depending on a dual income, and more men than ever before are filling the role of stay-at-home spouse and/or parent. Yet, so many men still skip out when it comes to making food for their families. Dialing up Domino's might technically count as "getting dinner on the table," but with a little more gumption, you can step up to the skillet and say, "I'm cooking dinner tonight." If you have kids, enlist your mini-chefs for simple tasks and enjoy your latest creation together at a table away from the TV. If this is not a regular occurrence in your house, expect to win major points with this move.

THE FUNDAMENTAL FIVE COOKING TECHNIQUES

Cooking is all about technique and timing. Technique can be taught, and timing comes with practice. When do you put the toast in the toaster so that it's still warm and toasty when your scrambled eggs are done? There are too many variables to give universal directions. So, we focus on technique, and know that your sense of timing will improve as you cook.

The fundamental five techniques you need to know for Refuel eating are:

1. Blend
2. Simmer
3. Grill
4. Roast
5. Stir-fry

ASSEMBLE WITH NOT SO MUCH CARE

Some days, the stove should not be turned on and the grill should be left alone. Maybe you just suffered through a brutal day at the office or the sweltering summer weather has made itself at home in your kitchen. Or, perhaps your wife and kids or roommates are off to the movies and you get to relish a quiet night at home. Or, maybe you've planned ahead and have foods in the fridge, freezer, or pantry that will combine well in a bowl or on a plate. These are the kinds of days that call for cook-free concoctions.

Check out more off-the-shelf recipes on page 205, but free-form meal assembly (when you are dealing with whatever's left in the fridge) works, too. Here are a couple ideas to get you thinking in the assembled-meal mindset:

1. Drain and rinse a can of black beans, then add Sriracha or your favorite hot sauce or salsa and chopped cilantro or sliced green onion.
2. Toss packaged mixed spring greens, diced avocado, and hard-cooked egg with a splash each of balsamic vinegar and olive oil. Add torn herbs such as basil, mint, chives, or thyme and top with freshly ground black pepper.
3. Mix refrigerated hummus (any flavor) with diced roasted chicken strips and a splash of lemon juice.
4. Shake a bagged salad into a bowl and rinse, then top with rotisserie chicken; add fresh dill, sliced cucumber, and sunflower seeds.
5. Choose grilled chicken or barbecue tempeh (a form of fermented soy that is dense like chicken breast) plus a broccoli hot dish from one part of the salad bar; top with toasted almonds and sunflower seeds in another (salad-bar meal; see more on salad-bar navigation on page 244).

> **MAN MEMO**
>
> Assembling foods is simply a matter of combining already prepared foods into a
> new dish. The formula is ABC:
>
> Acidic or spicy (lemon juice, vinegar, hot sauce), plus
> Bowl (bowl of something fresh, prepared or cooked), plus
> Crunch (any new texture—I like toasted seeds and crunchy
> vegetables)
>
> You've composed a quick and simple layered meal. Minimal cleanup required.

Blend

A high-quality blender, as described earlier in this chapter, will process ingredients at a speed of around 20,000 RPMs. In a matter of
seconds you can have the perfect juice, smoothie, soup, or salsa. Don't
try to substitute a food processor for a blender, since they perform
different functions. In general, food processors are better with dry ingredients; blenders are best for wet ingredients or those with a higher
water content.

You might think blending is a no-brainer, and for the most part
it is. But like anything else that involves extremely sharp blades spin-
ning at high speeds, smart strategies can come in handy. Also, always
disassemble a blender to clean its parts, which will prevent mold and
bacteria from developing, and try to return all parts to the same location after use. I like to have two blender jars, in case one is busy or
dirty, but this is not essential.

Ready to blend? Follow these "best blending practices," especially
when improvising a recipe:

- **Put the ingredients into the blender container before placing the container on
  the motor base.** The container is easier to reach when its bottom is on the counter or table, instead of on the motor base. Plus, you cut the risk of clotheslining
  the container and spilling its contents.
- **Add ingredients that need to be chopped first, with just a small amount of liquid.** A little liquid helps avoid cavitation, that invisible force field of air that

forms around the blades, preventing foods from actually blending. That little bubble blurp at the end? It's the blender farting. There is one exception to the solids-first rule: if you're using a higher-fat ingredient, such as full-fat coconut milk or heavy cream, add that first. You want the blade to whip air into it, foaming and giving volume to the liquid. (#blenderfart)

- **When it's hot, remove the top.** Mentioned earlier but bears repeating. When you add hot liquids to a blender, and you blend with the top on, steam will pressurize the container and it may blow the top off. It sounds funny, but it's not when the contents are hot. To prevent a hot mess, remove the lid center to let air escape and cover the opening with a folded towel before you start the motor.
- **Get into position.** Place your left thumb under the container handle and your four fingers atop the lid. Use your right hand to press the buttons. (If you are left-handed, switch left and right.) Give it a whir, leaving the top on 10 to 15 seconds to let the liquids settle and combine. Then buzz again, repeating as needed.
- **Motor control.** Like driving a car with a manual transmission, always start your blender in first gear, and then go up gradually. If you start in a higher gear, you can stall out the engine and end up with a sloppy consistency. Go up in a steplike fashion until the ingredients reach your desired consistency.
- **Know your level.** Try not to fill a blender container more than two-thirds full, ever. Spills happen.

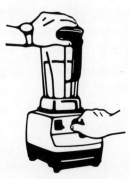

Blend responsibly: a topless blender will only lead to trouble.
Keep a lid on it, and you'll prevent messes.

Simmer

I love simmering because it melds flavors while preserving moistness.

Simmering, poaching, and boiling are all variations on the same method; they just happen at different points of temperature. Creating a simmer is an exercise in balancing a delicate tension—you heat the liquid until it moves and rises, but not to the point where it begins to bubble and actually break the surface.

> **CHEF'S SECRET**
>
> The temperature range for simmering at sea level is 180 to 200 degrees Fahrenheit. At 212 degrees at sea level, you've hit a boil (for every 500 feet in altitude, the boiling point drops by one degree): steady streams of large bubbles, followed by a raging torrent. You poach foods, such as eggs, at a lower temperature—between 160 and 180 degrees.

Boiling is good for beans, hard-cooked eggs, sweet potatoes, and lobsters—but carried on for a long time, it causes much more agitation and can break down other foods too far. To make sure you've hit the right temperature, grab an instant-read thermometer, which will tell you the temperature with just a quick dip. You can also look at the inside of the pot: if you see occasional large bubbles and a gently rumbling surface, you're at the right point.

To simmer, add the meat or vegetables you want to cook to the pot. Add cold liquid to cover. Turn on low to low-medium heat, and maintain the measured heat throughout the cooking process. Some meats, especially those injected with a cooking solution, foam when they simmer—a little protein floats to the surface: you can skim it or not.

Sounds pretty easy, right? It is. Simmering is not rocket science, but there are some tricks of the trade you can use to make standout food with this simple technique:

- **Use flavorful liquids.** You can simmer with water, but why miss this chance to create full-flavored food with a few added calories? Chicken or beef broth is great for stews; wines are for deepening pasta sauces; and juices add flavor to cuts of meat, such as corned beef, when cooked in apple juice and mustard.
- **The key to thickness is found in the lid.** With the lid off, any liquid in the pot will evaporate into the air and help concentrate the flavors—ideal when you're making a sauce. Keep the lid on when you're making grains and beans; you want them to absorb the cooking liquid, not the air.

- **Simmer, not slur.** When cooking with alcohol, keep the temperature above 180 degrees. Anything below that will not be hot enough to reduce or burn off the alcohol. While getting drunk from a dish might sound tempting, booze tastes much better in the glass.
- **Indirectly speaking.** Move the pot off of the direct heat if you're constantly fighting off a boil. This is especially useful when you're keeping a lid on the pot.
- **Frozen is just fine.** You can't roast frozen fish or vegetables very well, but you can simmer them. In fact, simmering frozen foods can help them retain moisture, especially frozen fish, like cod, halibut, and shellfish. Don't simmer them forever, though; cook just until opaque. Take the pan off the heat, taste, and serve.

Grill

There's nothing manlier than the combination of meat and fire. Toss a football in there and cue the Hemi engine soundtrack, and you might just shatter the scale of masculinity.

Now that we have the grilling stereotype out of the way, let's get to the technique. Whether it draws on some primitive instinct or not, there's no denying that grilling is a satisfying way to cook. It simply feels good to do it. It doesn't hurt that the flavors that come from a fire-hot grill can't truly be replicated any other way.

When it comes to grilling, the steps are simple: Get the grill hot. Place your foods on the grill, turning to cook both sides. Test for doneness and remove when ready. Within each of those steps there is plenty of room for interpretation, which means a wide-open opportunity for learning what to avoid and how to improve. Let's look at the dos and don'ts of grilling:

THE DOS OF GRILLING
- **Marinate your foods prior to grilling.** Marinades have three components: acid, oil, and aromatics. They add flavor and help to soften the surface of food, especially meats, and are best with foods that have relatively little fat: fish, hanger steak, boneless/skinless chicken breast, top sirloin/London broil, chicken thighs, and venison.

  Marinate at room temperature at your own risk: food spoils faster at room temperature than in the fridge. I recommend a maximum of an hour outside the fridge, and preferably less. A 1-gallon plastic bag is a great marinating vessel (no heat is involved, so you're not queuing up any estrogenic properties).

Make sure the food is covered with the marinade and flip the bag while it sits, so both sides absorb maximum flavor. If you can't stand wasting the extra marinade and have kept it constantly refrigerated, bring it to a boil and then simmer it for 5 minutes to turn it into a dipping sauce; it's tastier and more effective than basting. Increasing the surface area of all those flavor-rich ingredients means more on your meat, vegetables, and palate.

The flavor benefits to marinating are obvious, and marinades tenderize tougher cuts. Marinating will also cut your exposure to heterocyclic amines (HCAs), which are cancer-causing chemicals produced by grilling. Food chemists have found that marinating chicken in garlic, olive oil, and lemon juice for at least 15 minutes before grilling can cut levels of HCAs by 90 percent. With meats, a red wine or beer-based marinade for 6 hours can similarly cut HCAs by 90 percent. A rosemary and thyme oil-and-vinegar marinade for just 30 minutes did the same in an Oklahoma study. You can also minimize your exposure by cutting off charred bits before biting into grilled foods, and by grilling at low temperatures.

- **Dry-rub your fattiest cuts.** This doesn't work for vegetables, but they don't need it. Caribbean spices, Mediterranean mixtures, and plain old rosemary and thyme as dry rubs knock back cancer-causing chemicals like HCAs just as well as marinades. Use with fatty meats (an occasional treat), such as pork butt, duck, and brisket. You will create a crust that will change how you think about crust. The formula: fat + rub = crust.

▶ CHEF'S SECRET

Dry rubs are simpler than marinades: just spices and herbs. Still, it's important to make sure that you thoroughly press the spice mixture into the meat and that you use enough to go around, since rubs are all surface activity. Toast whole spices to kick up their flavor; it's a small step, but it pays you back, and with no extra calories.

- **Oil your grill.** First, clean the grill with a brush. While the grill is still cold, take a wadded-up paper towel and dip it in some oil. Wipe the grill down with the paper towel (using your tongs). You only need a little bit; too much will spark flare-ups.
- **Treat your meat with respect.** Don't just slap it on the grill. Use a backhand grip to roll steak, chicken, or a fillet of fish onto the grill; do so at a 45-degree angle if you want extra-special grill marks. Line up the items in orderly fashion,

because it just looks nice and it will help you keep track of the order in which you put foods on the grill.

- **Demand sizzle.** Hold your hand 3 inches above the grill: if it's hot enough, you'll have to take it away in under 3 seconds. When you roll your food onto the grill, you should hear the sweet sound of sizzle. If you don't, remove your food and wait until the grill is hotter.

THE DON'TS OF GRILLING

- **Turn meat more than once.** Turning often only toughens up the tissue. Grill on one side until you see a little moisture on top, then flip over.
- **Pour marinade on food while it's cooking.** This is probably the most common grilling mistake. When you pour marinade directly onto foods on the grill, you don't add moisture or flavor or tenderize; you only increase the chances of flare-ups. If you can't resist, paint little amounts of marinade onto the food, but even that can have little effect.
- **Pack the house.** Leave room for your foods to cook evenly and for you to turn them: leave at least 2 inches between items.
- **Prematurely maul your foods.** Cutting into meat while it's still on the grill can undo all your efforts to create a satisfying steak. A premature slice will not only dry out meats, it will also make them look unattractive. Instead, use the Tongs & Touch Test (see sidebar below) or an instant-read thermometer.
- **Mash your meat or veg.** Mashing means dried-out meals that don't cook any faster. Avoid the temptation.

▶ TONGS & TOUCH TEST

Here's a simple, consistent way to check the temperature of grilled meats:

Rare: Make a circle with your index finger and thumb. With the index finger from your opposite hand, press the ball on the palm side of your thumb—it should feel very soft. Now, press the center of your steak with tongs or your finger. If the textures match, your steak is rare.

Medium rare: Make a circle with your middle finger and thumb. Press the ball of your thumb again; this is medium rare.

Medium: Make a circle with your ring finger and thumb. Check ball of thumb. When this texture matches your steak's, you've hit medium.

Well done: Press your little finger and thumb together—the ball of your thumb should feel very firm; this is what a well-done steak feels like.

Roast

Did you know you could roast an apple pie and bake a pork tenderloin? That's because roasting and baking are the same technique; we just use the terms differently depending on what's being cooked. When you roast (or bake) foods, you use dry heat to cook foods from the outside in. This is why, if you cook something at the wrong temperature, you can have a well-done exterior and undercooked interior—that's dangerous with some cuts of meat and unsavory with others. It's also why when you roast foods the key elements to keep in mind are temperature and time.

Unless you're roasting a wild boar on a spit or a pig in a fire pit, roasting technique is as simple as it comes. If you have an oven and something on which to place your ingredients, you can be a top-notch roaster. I like to think of it as the Lay-Z-Boy of cooking methods since the oven does almost all the work.

For this reason, I suggest making sure that what your oven tells you is true—inaccurate temperature gauges can drastically throw off your cooking outcomes. You can recalibrate your oven, but this can be a tedious process. Another option is to place an oven thermometer on one side of the oven, and a second one on the other side to take accurate readings. If the readings match your oven's temp, you can take the gauges out; if not, leave them in and use their readings as your cooking temperature.

As in grilling, there are specific dos and don'ts that apply when roasting foods.

THE DOS OF ROASTING

- **Bring to room temperature.** Remove the meats and poultry (especially boneless items) from the refrigerator 15 to 20 minutes prior to placing them in the oven. Letting them warm to room temperature will ensure consistency and more dependable cooking times. While not critical, it's a good habit to get into.

- **Match entree to vessel size.** A roast should not spill over the sides of a meat-loaf tin, nor should a solo quail rest in a 12-gallon pot. Place a rib roast or tenderloin in a sizable roasting pan with at least 2-inch sides to contain the juices. Vegetables can go on a shallow sheet pan lined with parchment paper (if you have it). Using the right-size vessel allows you to leave some space around the foods you're cooking. When working with multiples of any ingredient, be sure to spread them out in a single layer and try to avoid overlap.
- **Ask yourself two questions.** Before placing a pan in the oven, ask yourself: Is the oven hot? Check the temperature reading and if it's not ready, wait. Is there fat in what I'm roasting? Fat helps prevent foods from drying out. Most meat has plenty of natural fat for roasting, but vegetables should get lubed in olive oil—up to about 1 teaspoon per cup of veggies. Nuts and seeds also have their own fat, but don't skimp on the seasoning. Kosher salt, white and black pepper, paprika, and some salt-free spice mixes (I like Mrs. Dash, and the custom blends of thespicehouse.com and of penzeys.com) all add a nice pop of flavor to roasted nuts.

THE DON'TS OF ROASTING

- **Fill your kitchen with toxic fumes.** Do not use nonstick pans for roasting (or for any other method that uses high heat, such as stir-frying). When nonstick pans reach a temperature of 680 degrees, according to EWG.org tests of Teflon, pans begin to emit a number of toxic gases into the air; toxic particles begin at 464 degrees. Perfluorooctanoic acid, also known as PFOA or C-8, is also released; it's a probable carcinogen, according to EPA scientists, and appears to raise cholesterol and may contribute to ADHD in children. Use a stainless-steel or ceramic-lined cast-iron Dutch oven, a stainless-steel roasting pan, or a stainless-steel or ceramic casserole dish.
- **Feel the need to baste.** Basting is overrated—it lowers the temperature of the oven (since you have to keep it open while basting) and changes the temperature of what you're cooking.
- **Skip the resting stage.** Remove meats and dense vegetables from the oven, place on a platter or cutting board with a rim to catch the juices, and cover with aluminum foil for 10 minutes before slicing. The muscle fibers in a piece of meat constrict when cooked, which makes them less capable of absorption. Once removed from heat, they cool and open up, soaking up succulent juices like a sponge. Have you ever cut into a nice steak and woefully watched all the juice spill onto your plate or cutting board? Chances are it just needed more rest.

- **Carve with the grain.** Like a piece of wood, meat has a grain that comes from the natural structure of its fibers. In certain cuts of meat, like flank, hanger, and skirt steak, these fibers can be dense and tight rows of muscle. If you cut parallel to these rows, you keep the integrity of the fibers intact, creating a tough and chewy bite. Before even taking a bite, you can tell meat has been cut with the grain if it is in long strips with lines that run with the natural lines of the meat. It's easy to cut against the grain if you pay attention. Slice into a piece of meat or poultry and take a good look at it—the grain of the meat should run perpendicular to the cut of your knife. Feel free to test the tenderness of the bite.

Stir-Fry

Stir-frying is all about creating fast, flavorful one-pot meals using high heat. It's a great technique because it can be relatively forgiving—with the right ingredients all in one pot, how bad could it possibly turn out? Here, the worst you can do is overcook the vegetables until they're mushy—not great, but still edible. (Of course, you should aim higher than just to create edible meals, but it's a starting point.)

Let's look at the most notable dos and don'ts of stir-frying.

THE DOS OF STIR-FRYING

- **Strategically prepare.** The most important part of stir-frying is preparation. You should have all your ingredients prepped and ready when you turn on the stovetop. Everything happens so fast that it will be hard to catch up if you don't.
- **Same type = same size.** Prep ingredients so that foods are the same general size and shape. Vegetables should be cut into 1- or 2-inch pieces and proteins (fish, meat, poultry, tofu, tempeh, seitan) should be sliced into chunks or sections that will be easy to eat in one or two bites.
- **Follow the rule of density.** When making a stir-fry dish, let density tell the cooking times. For example, broccoli is firm and fibrous and will take 3 to 4 minutes to soften, cook, and brighten in color; sturdy leafy greens such as bok choy will take less than 3 minutes; paper-thin spinach takes just a few seconds. No need to memorize this—you will learn with practice.
- **Tumble the ingredients.** Grace Young is the master of stir-fries, and I think this is her most important tip (and she has many other great ones, too). Tumbling lets the ingredients briefly and evenly touch the bottom of the hot flat-bottomed wok, and doesn't force them to disintegrate, as over-stirring may.

> **CHEF'S SECRET**
> Using an electric stove? Light up two burners at a time, keeping one on low heat and the other on high. Then, just move your pan from one to the other as needed.

THE DON'TS OF STIR-FRYING

- **Oil the pan or wok.** Ah, the sound of the sizzle . . . it's great until the scalding spray of oil comes splashing up on your bare skin or shirt. Instead of adding all the cooking oil to a hot pan, coat the meat or vegetables in oil before dropping them in. This will also ensure that everything gets a full coat of flavor.
- **Cook one ingredient at a time.** Authentic stir-fry technique requires that each ingredient be cooked and then removed. At the end, they're all added together so the flavors can meld. It's not worth your time unless you're going for perfection—in which case, be my guest and go for it. But the first time around, try cooking the densest ingredients first and the least dense last. This shortcut will create quicker, more satisfying, and practical meals. Just stick to the rule of density and you and any hungry eaters for whom you're cooking will be justly delighted.
- **Add meats first.** Instead, save the meat, poultry, seafood, and tofu for near the end. They will cook quickly and stay tender if you do this.
- **Pour in the center of the pan.** Instead, pour in any liquid you're adding along the sides of the pan. This will ensure that the liquid doesn't soak the middle and turn the stir-fry into a stew, as well as lower the temperature of the whole dish. You want crisp, fresh bites from a stir-fry, not soggy ones.
- **Overdose on the rice.** Yes, I know this isn't a technique. But rice is often thought to be the foundation of the stir-fry once plated. It doesn't have to be and shouldn't be. Brown rice or wild rice, heavily larded with dried mushrooms and a few sun-dried tomatoes and touched with soy sauce, is perfect with a stir-fry: and you need about $1/2$ cup of cooked rice per 6-inch plate.

A MARATHON, NOT A SPRINT

Approach cooking as you would any other skill: you must practice and train to see improvement. Learn to slice, dice, and chop with a chef's knife that feels good in your hand. The recipes in chapter 14 will awaken your metabolic advantages and manly cooking skills.

SEE, TASTE, EAT

Fridge, Pantry, and Freezer Must-Haves

Hunger is a biological urge, hunting for food is primal, and eating sustains life. Men eat what they find in the environment. Prehistoric men found foods like meats, fish, roots, and berries. Today's men find Big Macs, double-stuffed Oreos, chili cheese fries, and fried chicken—and whatever's in the fridge at eye level. No wonder you're overweight. You've been drugged.

You could eat like a caveman to snap out of the stupor, regain energy and stamina, and lose the gut. You could live in a cave to find a better environment. There's a lot of appeal to the cave, and the fire, and the loin skin. And the whole primal, paleo way of eating.

In the modern world of changing family dynamics, get-togethers after work, and the church social, however, it's tough to pull off the caveman thing 24/7—and not good for your teeth.

Fortunately, you are a product of thousands of years of evolution—there's no reason you should have to go backward to move forward. With knowledge and practice, you can deploy smart NOG™ (nuggets of gold) strategies to find the hidden gems in whatever environment you find yourself in. When done right, these strategies effectively establish automatic behaviors in your home, at the office, or on the go. To accomplish this, you must outfit your environment with the foods you need to lose the gut. It's simple: you plan and prepare.

> ### CUE CONTROL

We all have a primal response to food. The smell, sound, taste, and texture trigger neurological and metabolic fireworks. How this works differs between men and women.

When researchers at the University of Oregon tempted hungry men and women with their favorite foods, the men could shut off their brain's response while the women couldn't. Here's the setup: foods like pizza, bacon-egg-and-cheese sandwiches, and fried chicken were warmed so their aromas wafted into the room full of study participants. Samples of the flavors were dabbed on their tongues. And then researchers measured the participants' brain pleasure centers for activity.

When men applied cognitive inhibition—ignoring or shifting their thoughts away from the smells and lingering tastes—they could shut off those pleasure centers. Women didn't have this override ability to the same extent. The takeaway is this: you can flex your brain muscles to crush any habits of impulsive eating.

HOW YOU CAN AVOID THE TRAP OF JUNK FOOD, TV DINNERS, AND SALTY, FATTY, CHEAP TAKEOUT

You may have heard of the Standard American Diet (SAD). The acronym is silly, conveying emotion instead of a physical consequence; Generally Ubiquitous Toxins (GUT) would be more appropriate.

Pushers of SAD are posted on nearly every corner in most American cities. The reality is that the food environment in which we all live does not cater to your best interests. SAD purveyors do not care about your high cholesterol, your borderline diabetes, your muscle mass, or your erectile ability.

Bottom line: you can't depend on the environment around you to provide the foods you need to lose your gut and boost your T. Be a man in control by setting up shop appropriately and efficiently. That is, shop with a plan and practice safe snacking.

THE GROCERY STORE PLAYBOOK

Losing your gut depends on getting the right foods into your house. Since surveys have shown that up to 51 percent of men are now the primary grocery shoppers in their households, many men are directly involved in what goes into the fridge, pantry, and freezer. If this is you, the playbook will be a simple process of implementation. If you're not one of those guys, and you don't plan to become one, share this chapter with your wife, girlfriend, or partner (maybe along with some flowers or a handwritten card).

First ground rule: unless you develop a real passion for food, shopping for it should not become a hobby. Go to buy, not to shop. The mindset should be "get in, get what's mine, get on with my life." Sounds easy, but it's not always. There are processed-food companies out there fighting tooth and nail for your hard-earned dollar. And they will stalk you through the aisles, tempting you with slogans, packaging, car-size displays, and deals. How do you avoid being their prey? A few ways:

1. **Go with a list or commit to memory your staple goods.** You can use the Refuel shopping lists, or you can create your own. You can also shop straight from a recipe, new or favorite. If it's a favorite, chances are its flavors suit your palate. Stock up on those same ingredients and spices, and use them in new ways as you build more confidence in the kitchen.
2. **Pack your cart with produce first.** This sets the tone for the trip. With a cart half full of fresh goods, you'll be less likely to toss in nutrient zombies—highly processed items like packaged cookies, chips, candy bars, and frozen mini taquitos. Really, dude? Mini taquitos?
3. **Never hit the aisles hungry.** Sage advice worth repeating. Even drinking a big glass of water beforehand can help curb impulse buys.

▶ I'M HEADING OUT TO PICK UP SOME NUTRITION—WANT ANYTHING?

Competitive athletes view food as fuel that stokes biologic and metabolic functions. Just as we know most cars won't run without gas, athletes know their bodies will sputter out without proper nutrition. They ask: "What makes me perform at my best?"

The noncompetitive athletes among us can take our cues from this mindset. Eat with purpose and with a goal in mind. Pleasure counts as a goal—that's a given. But I mean a goal you can measure and see. Record your progress and performance, and you'll move closer to your goal.

Another common strategy for smart shopping is worth noting, if only because it's no longer entirely accurate. Many smart nutritionists and food experts have recommended that all shopping be done along the perimeter of the grocery store. The suggestion was based on the marketing practice of placing the fresh, whole foods, such as produce, dairy, and meats, along the edges of the store. But brands and stores have outsmarted this recommendation. Today you'll find processed foods next to the whole fruits and vegetables or meats. The new rule is this: explore the perimeter, be wary, and shop from the plan, knowing what foods will produce the results you want.

The foods that will boost your T and help you drop belly fat are in the list that follows. Create a "Man Shelf" in your pantry and also in the fridge and freezer—these places are where the food you're going to eat will now live.

REFUEL SHELF STAPLES	
COUNTERTOP GOODS	
apples	garlic
avocados	lemons
cherry tomatoes	onions
citrus fruits	

PANTRY ESSENTIALS

beef broth, reduced sodium, canned

black beans, canned, no salt added

brown rice

chickpeas, canned

coffee

cornstarch

dark sesame oil*

high-protein, high-fiber cereal

hot sauce*

jerky (beef, bison, salmon, and turkey)

kidney beans, canned, no salt added

lentils

light unsweetened coconut milk, canned*

mustard (Dijon and spicy brown)*

natural peanut butter

olive oil

onions

oysters, smoked or canned

quinoa

salsa, jarred*

sardines, canned

soup cups, shelf-stable

soy sauce, reduced sodium

steel-cut oats

stevia

tomatoes, diced, canned

tuna in water, canned

unsweetened cocoa

vegetable broth, canned

vinegar, apple cider

whey powder

wine, red*

Worcestershire sauce

FRIDGE FAVORITES

asparagus spears

basil, fresh

beef chuck stew meat, boneless, grass-fed

broccoli

cabbage, green and red

carrots

cauliflower

celery

chicken breasts and thighs

cilantro

cottage cheese

cucumbers

eggs, cage-free or omega-3 rich

hummus

jicama

kale

lemon juice concentrate, Santa Cruz organic

lemons

lettuce

light sour cream

mushrooms, button

Parmigiano-Reggiano cheese

parsley, Italian

salsa, fresh

sirloin steak, boneless, grass-fed

smoked salmon

tofu in water, firm

turkey, ground, 93% fat-free

yogurt, Greek-style

* Refrigerate after opening

FREEZER PERENNIALS

almonds	pistachios in the shell
berries, mixed	pumpkin seeds
burgers, bison*	semisweet or bittersweet chocolate
burgers, salmon	chips
burgers, veggie	squash seeds
cashews	walnuts
edamame	watermelon seeds, toasted
fish (salmon, tuna, halibut, mahimahi:	whole chickens, 3–4 pounds*
whatever is fresh and on sale)*	whole turkey or chicken breasts*
pecans	

SPICE RACK

black pepper, ground	onion salt
chili powder, salt-free	oregano
cinnamon, ground	poultry seasoning
crushed red pepper flakes	rosemary
garlic salt	sea salt
jerk seasonings	sesame seeds, toasted
kosher salt	thyme
Mediterranean spice mix, salt-free	

*Can be bought fresh or frozen

THE SCIENCE OF SEEING

Better organization and better planning will lead to better eating and help you win, with simplicity and effectiveness, the war being waged against you in the food environment (i.e., from your doorway to the office to the store and back, and sometimes in your very own kitchen, den, or man cave). This means—in the most controllable of these environments, your kitchen—putting the testosterone-boosting foods in your sightlines and relegating the processed, estrogen-inducing foods to the lower ranks or even discharging them altogether.

The first step is to survey the territory. Like the game of Clue, you'll try to find what's killing your energy and sex drive, and sabotaging your muscle-building abilities. Take a look around your house and ask yourself two questions:

1.   Where do I go when I'm hungry?
2.   What do I find there?

The question then becomes, What if instead of cookies, chips, and beer I were to find lean-muscle-mass-producing, belly-fat-burning foods there? Certainly the chances that you would choose them increase greatly.

▶ THE BIKINI BEER CONNECTION

Most of us have a nice collection of automatic behaviors. For example, when you sit in your favorite chair after work, do you find it impossible not to grab a beer?

You can condition yourself to have a more productive habit. Place your sneakers or something relaxing to read just where you will see them as you walk in the door from work. Then, challenge yourself: walk in those sneakers, or read that magazine article—or do pushups or put on headphones and listen to music for 10 minutes before you do anything else. A quick decompression session will channel that autopilot behavior into something better than the calories you don't need before you sit down to dinner.

The obvious way to override reflexive eating is to avoid bringing those belly-fat-boosting foods into the house in the first place. Alternatively, you can outsmart the indulgence by making your Refuel foods the most visible ones:

- **On the Counter:** Use a brightly colored bowl and in it place small apples and citrus fruits.
- **In the Fridge:** The shelves that are eye level are most important. Fill a pitcher with citrus water and store it on the top shelf. Place slices of fresh vegetables in glass containers where you can see them. Foods like red pepper slices and hummus should catch your eye before that gargantuan container of macaroni salad. Why is that tub of starch and glop there anyway?

- **In the Pantry:** Keep pre-portioned bags of nuts, seeds, trail mix, and high-protein cereal in a basket, ready for a quick grab. Stock your glove compartment, your laptop bag, your desk drawer with these snacks (see page 203 for ideas). If you buy items in bulk, always break them down and store them in smaller portions. According to Brian Wansink (introduced in Chapter 7), "When you buy in bulk, you eat in bulk." For obvious reasons, bulk eating should be avoided.

Remember: Visibility is king. Put the foods you want to eat where you will see them. I know this may sound second-grade simple. And the strategy *is*, but the science behind it is based on human behavior, which is as complicated and messy as it gets.

> **HOT TIP**
>
> Refueled men prefer nuts for snacking. Strategies for avoiding prolonged snacking include eating three full meals daily, drinking citrus water, and exercising instead of eating.

ATTACK OF THE SNACK(S)

Fewer sit-down meals and fast-paced lifestyles have made snacks a mainstay of today's eating. There's nothing inherently wrong with having a snack or, at most, two to get you through the day, but current habits have some serious flaws:

1. **Snacking should not be an ongoing action or a hobby.** Think of it as a noun ("I ate a snack"), not a verb ("I'm snacking"). When you have a snack, consider it a delicious moment to savor, and sustenance with which you can stave off hunger for a few hours until you can have a satisfying meal.
2. **It's not dessert, a meal, or a carb-athon.** A twenty-year study of 120,000 people called out the potato chip as the single biggest factor related to weight gain (more potato chips consumed, more pounds put on). Not so coincidentally, the most commonly consumed snack in the United States is the potato chip. When you snack on foods that lack protein, good fats, or fiber, you set the stage for fat storage, followed by overeating.

Highly processed and refined carbohydrates (especially added sugar) dump nearly straight into your bloodstream as glucose. This promotes a surge of insulin, which works frantically to move glucose into the cells. When your muscles are full of fuel, which is most of the time except after a strenuous workout, insulin will bypass the muscle cells and stimulate the conversion of glucose into fat so it can be stored in fat cells for future use. When your glucose levels come crashing down, you feel like you want to inhale the contents of the vending machine even though you just ate. So, step away from the potato chips, and no one will get hurt.

> ## ▶ HOT TIP
> Thirty percent of people given a 100-calorie snack pack ate more than when they were given a larger serving from which to eat. Pay attention, or better yet, skip these snack traps altogether: most 100-calorie snack packs contain processed, crushable foods (exception is nuts).

Snacks are not meals. Because there's often no sense of relief from hunger, people recall a snack as being much less calorie dense than it actually is. Adding 2 minutes (or 2 hours) of walking to your exercise does not compensate for two "snack-size" bags of Doritos and three Chips-Ahoy cookies—even if you barely remember eating them.

> ## ▶ THE HIGH PRICE OF A SNACK
> When you have to rely on a vending machine for food, select the nuts, trail mix, jerky, or any kind of canned tuna, chicken, or salmon. Should you get shorted on change, or find you can't reach your snack pack, skip the wrestling match with the 800-pound gorilla that vends. It's not worth it. And take it as a sign!

On Refuel, the snack can stay, but a strategic approach is critical. I've outlined three steps to smart snack selection. Notably, the sodium suggestion will be the toughest to follow—when and if you can't meet this measure, be diligent with hydration throughout the day to help flush out the extra salt.

The Three-Step Guide to Picking Smart Snacks

I. Opt for items that have more protein and fiber added together than total carbs. Keep sugar to less than 6 grams.

2. Skip high-sodium items when possible; 250 milligrams or less per serving you actually eat is ideal.

3. Grab foods with fewer ingredients over those with long lists of items you don't know how to pronounce. Less really is more sometimes.

Timing is important to consider here, too—is it truly time to fuel? Or is it less than two hours before or after a meal? If so, stop eating and switch to citrus water.

Snacking can easily become a brainless activity, subconsciously continuing while you work, watch TV, or drive a car. Even healthy-fat, protein-packed snacks should not be eaten to the point where they become or replace a meal.

At work, instead of keeping snacks right on your desk, stock a few Ziploc bags of nonperishable foods in a drawer so that you have to get up and walk to them. Research done at the Cornell Food and Brand Lab found that if people had to walk just 6 feet from their desk, they ate more than 50 percent less than if an item was within arm's reach. You don't have to create an obstacle course between you and a snack; the simple act of standing up and taking a few steps is enough to prevent dazed-out grazing.

TOP 40 SNACKS FOR MEN

Here are a total of forty specific ideas for snacks, many of which you can easily pack in your laptop bag or gym duffel—no vending machine required. Check labels for important details: look for "unsweetened," "no nitrates and nitrites," and "high fiber." Even better, look for no packaging: fresh is best. Avoid foods with the "fat free" label: these items are usually pumped full of sugar to make up for loss of flavor. Look for dairy that is modest in fat and, in small quantities, full fat. Rarely can nonfat dairy products deliver very good flavor; reduced-fat and full-fat items, on the other hand, satiate in smaller quantities. The best snacks have less than 200 calories.

Fridge and Freezer Snacks

1. Fresh sliced vegetables: bell peppers, carrots, celery, cucumbers, cherry or grape tomatoes, mushrooms, broccoli, cauliflower, jicama, radishes (unlimited)
2. Chobani, Athenos, or FAGE plain Greek yogurt with chopped walnuts (1 cup)
3. Hummus made with tahini (2 tablespoons)
4. Classic Protein Guy Shake (page 209)
5. Cottage cheese: sweet with fresh fruit or savory with chopped tomato, salt, and pepper ($\frac{1}{2}$ cup)
6. Hard-cooked eggs (up to 2)
7. Avocado and cucumber salad with rice wine vinegar (1 cup)
8. Slices of cold roasted chicken or turkey breast or grilled lean steak (1–2 ounces)
9. Salmon burger (1)
10. Raspberries, blackberries, blueberries, and strawberries (1 cup)
11. String cheese (1 ounce)
12. Laughing Cow blue cheese (2 wedges)
13. Mini Babybel cheese (2 rounds)
14. Smoked salmon (1–2 ounces)
15. Cherry tomatoes and mozzarella bites ($\frac{1}{4}$ cup)

▶ CHEF'S SECRETS

Fresh jicama is crisp, sweet, and refreshing. The trick is in knowing how to prepare it. It's simple if you follow these steps:

1. Cut the top and bottom ends off with a sharp knife. This will give you a stable cutting surface.
2. Peel off the outer skin with a potato peeler or carefully remove with your knife. You want to remove all of the thick rind.
3. Rinse peeled jicama and slice or cube based on your preference. I prefer it in triangles: make rough slices, and then cut into triangles. Better for guacamole.

Power Pantry Snacks

16. Roasted or raw almonds: 100-calorie packs or buy bulk bags of raw almonds and roast at home and pre-portion: count out 23 almonds per bag (1 ounce)

17. Pistachios in the shell: raw or roasted with spices (1 ounce, about 47 nuts)

18. Roasted or raw pumpkin, squash, and sunflower seeds (1 ounce)

19. Kale chips (1 ounce)

20. Popcorn: add paprika, chili powder, fresh-grated parmesan (butter spray is okay, but watch the amount) (1 cup)

21. Chunk light tuna in water or oil in a pouch or can (3 ounces)

22. Bumble Bee Premium Wild Pink Salmon Pouch (3 ounces)

23. Organic peanut butter or almond butter (1–2 teaspoons) spread on celery

24. Oatmeal: steel-cut with walnuts, made with almond or rice milk ($\frac{1}{2}$ cup)

25. Small apples (plain or with peanut or almond butter)

26. Green tea with or without honey or stevia or orange slice

27. Smoked oysters or baby clams in olive oil ($\frac{1}{2}$ can)

28. Sardines with lemon on dense whole-grain crackers or rusks (6 crackers) with red pepper flakes

29. Canned artichoke hearts in water or oil, with feta and oregano ($\frac{1}{2}$ cup)

30. 1 ounce of hard cheese, such as Manchego, aged Gouda, Romano, and Parmigiano

31. One or two softer cheese sticks, such as mozzarella and Cheddar: tear into strings for more surface area

32. Unsweetened turkey or salmon jerky, up to 4 ounces

33. Cup of lentil, vegetable, or black bean soup, such as Right Foods Black Bean and Lime

34. Seaweed chips (10–20 chips)

35. Tangerines, tangelos, small grapefruit, small orange

36. Cacao nibs (1 ounce), from Scharffen Berger

37. Dark chocolate–covered almonds (1 ounce)

Make Your Own Snacks

38. **Homemade Quick Pickles:** Simmer 1 cup cider vinegar, 2 teaspoons salt, and 3 bay leaves just until the salt is dissolved. Place 4 cups sliced cucumbers and 2 tablespoons chopped fresh dill (optional but good) in a

large bowl, and add the vinegar mixture. Store in the fridge. Ready in 24 hours. Unlimited portion.

39. **Two-Bean Salad:** Rinse a l5-ounce can of chickpeas and a l5-ounce can of black beans. Add half a diced red onion, and red wine vinegar, olive oil, and salt and pepper to taste. A portion is $\frac{1}{2}$ cup.

40. **Refuel Trail Mix:** It's all about texture, so go for some crunchy ingredients, some soft, and some in between. My favorite mix is $\frac{1}{3}$ cup raw almonds; $\frac{1}{3}$ cup toasted pistachios, squash seeds, or watermelon seeds; $\frac{1}{3}$ cup raw walnuts; and one Brazil nut for a boost of selenium. A portion is one small handful.

▶ THE SUPER SNACK YOU'RE NOT EATING

If you frequently dine on sushi, you've probably tried seaweed salad. This fresh-tasting, bright green condiment is an often-overlooked nutrient powerhouse.

Seaweed is rich in magnesium, calcium, iodine, and folate. More remarkable is its high concentration of anti-aging molecules called fucoidans, which are thought to be a key contributor to the extraordinary rates of longevity in Japan. Fucoidans help protect and regenerate tissue and organs, inhibit photo-aging of skin (resulting from UV rays), boost immune health, and fight against bacteria, viruses, and certain types of cancer. It's also chock-full of starchy phycocolloids that aid in the removal of heavy metals such as cadmium, arsenic, and lead.

Look for seaweed in the form of salads and chips, the latter of which can be found at Trader Joe's and Costco in small, single-serving packs.

A PRODUCT OF YOUR OWN ENVIRONMENT

The most visible foods in your home and office are the ones you're most likely to eat first. Then, eventually you'll see what you eat manifest itself in another form (no, not just in the toilet, but in the mirror, too).

Consistently choosing snacks rich in protein and high-quality foods over refined, highly processed sugary varieties will help keep the wrong hormones suppressed, promote lean muscle building, and accelerate belly-fat loss. You will see and feel the difference.

14

SURVIVAL MEALS FOR MEN

15 Dishes Every Man Should Know How to Make

Most people make cooking too complicated. You don't need culinary future science or a talking refrigerator to cook. Focus on gathering fresh ingredients first, and you'll immediately prioritize flavor and fat loss.

For me, cooking is control. I get to use knives; I get to work with fire; I get to produce something tangible, beautiful, and tasty. On my terms. I hope you challenge yourself to practice and perfect a minimum of one recipe from this chapter. (Citrus water and hard-cooked eggs do not count.)

So it's time to man the kitchen. If you're new to cooking, make it simple by starting with a shake and working up to a steak.

CITRUS WATER

Technique: Assemble
Tools: Chef's knife
Preparation time: 5 minutes
Servings: 12

I ask my patients to make an effort to carry citrus water with them wherever they go; if they're based at home, they also keep a supply in the fridge. If you've had trouble drinking enough water in the past, the citrus kick should help you get into the right way to hydrate. The benefits go beyond taste—citrus juice has been shown to help stimulate fat loss, improve muscle performance, and reduce fatigue. German scientists found that drinking 16 ounces upon waking can provide an extra metabolic burst. So wake up, and then drink up: 3 liters, every day.

One other note: the juice is strong. It's meant to remind you that you are drinking something. If it's too strong, you can cut back on the lemon juice. But remember to drink all 3 liters daily. It's essential.

> 3 liters (about 12 cups) filtered water (see Tips)
> I tangerine or small orange, preferably organic, washed and quartered (optional)
> ¾ cup fresh or bottled lemon or lime juice; if bottled, preferably Santa Cruz organic brand

1. Combine the water, fruit (if using), and juice in a covered large glass container; stir well.
2. Keep refrigerated up to 2 days.
3. Drink all in one day.

TIPS: Try a pitcher with a filter for your citrus water: remove the lid and filter from your filtered water, stir in the fruit and juice, and store in the refrigerator. Drink the water with meals and also take to the gym or to work, transferring it to a BPA-free water bottle. Thermos brand makes a stainless-steel water bottle with a single-handed flip top that keeps the water chilled for hours.

You can use just the juice and strain out the fruit or add the quartered fruit to the juice mixture. Experiment to see which concentration of citrus you prefer.

Zinger Water: Add ½ cup dried hibiscus blossoms and sepals or 3 hibiscus tea bags to 3 liters of filtered water. Steep overnight and then drink. Try the Republic of Tea's selection of tea bags.

NUTRITIONAL INFORMATION PER SERVING
Calories: 3 • Protein: 0 g • Fat: 0 g • Carbohydrates: I g • Sugar: 0 g • Total fiber: I g • Sodium: 0 mg

CLASSIC PROTEIN GUY SHAKE, THREE WAYS

Technique: Blend
Tools: Blender
Preparation time: 10 minutes
Servings: 1 (about 1¼ cups per serving)

Not a shake kind of guy? You will be after you try this version with coconut milk, which gives your new favorite drink (yes, I'm that confident you'll love it) a smooth, rich base. The Classic Protein Guy Shake became a staple morning meal for most of my Refuel success stories.

A 6-ounce (¾ cup) serving of Greek yogurt will enhance the texture while providing 17 grams of protein. If you're a big fan of protein powder, check out the variation below. Look for protein powder that's an isolate rather than a concentrate—the former blends better and is lower in carbohydrates and fat.

¾ cup 2% low-fat plain Greek yogurt
¼ cup frozen unsweetened mixed berries, not thawed
¼ cup light coconut milk (see Tip)
1 tablespoon flaxseed meal
1 packet stevia sweetener, such as Pyure
½ teaspoon ground cinnamon
¼ cup crushed ice or 2 large ice cubes

1. Combine the yogurt, frozen berries, coconut milk, flaxseed meal, sweetener, and cinnamon in the blender container.
2. Cover; blend until fairly smooth, about 10 seconds.
3. Add the ice cubes; cover and blend 10 seconds more. The shake will be thick. For a thinner shake, add a little water. For a very thick shake, add more ice cubes.

TIP: Transfer any leftover coconut milk from the can to a glass jar and refrigerate up to 4 days. Shake well before using.

SUBSTITUTIONS: Frozen raspberries or blackberries may replace the mixed fruit, and pumpkin pie spice or apple pie spice may replace the cinnamon.

NUTRITIONAL INFORMATION PER SERVING (MASTER RECIPE)
Calories: 222 • Protein: 19 g • Fat: 10 g • Carbohydrates: 17 g • Sugar: 11 g •
Total fiber: 4 g • Sodium: 75 mg

Strawberry Vanilla Shake (Vegan): Substitute 10 ounces silken lite tofu for the yogurt, frozen unsweetened strawberries for the mixed berries, and 1 teaspoon vanilla extract for the cinnamon. Yields 1¾ cups. (Calories: 191, protein: 20 g, fat: 4 g, carbs: 8 g, sugar: 2 g, total fiber: 3 g, sodium: 213 mg)

Raspberry Chocolate Shake (with protein powder): Substitute ½ cup unsweetened almond milk (such as Silk brand) plus 1 scoop (⅓ cup) Jay Robb or Now brand chocolate-flavored whey powder or egg white powder for the yogurt and coconut milk; use frozen unsweetened raspberries instead of the mixed berries; and add 1 teaspoon unsweetened cocoa powder instead of the cinnamon. Omit the stevia, and increase the ice to ½ cup. Yields 1¼ cups. (Calories: 180, protein: 28 g, fat: 4 g, carbs: 8 g, sugar: 1 g, total fiber: 4 g, sodium: 241 mg)

> **THE SILKY WAY**
>
> Silken tofu is undrained tofu, and that extra water content allows you to whip a shake into great shape. If you're concerned about modest soy consumption and your manhood, you shouldn't be. A 2010 meta-analysis of soy studies revealed that soy foods did not alter sex hormones in men, and additional research has shown that soy products have no effect on sperm quality.

FOOLPROOF HARD-COOKED EGGS

Technique: Boil/simmer
Tools: Dutch oven or large saucepan
Preparation time: 30 minutes
Servings: 12 (2 eggs per serving)

Like cooking rice or boiling a perfect potato, hard-cooking eggs can be an exercise in disappointment—the technique seems deceptively simple, yet miscalculations on cooking time and water measurement can lead to trouble. You can end up with runny whites, chalky yolks, or brittle bits of shell that frustrate you as you peel the eggs.

The formula for success is one part cooking time, one part ingredient selection, and one part proper cooldown. You'll notice the direct cooking time is minimal; the passive heat in the water is enough to slow-cook the eggs through to their yolk centers.

As for the star ingredient, it's best to work with eggs that are slightly older—this isn't Hollywood. The membrane lining the fresh egg shell will pull away from the shell, given a bit of time. This makes peeling a much simpler process, giving you bigger breakaway pieces rather than stubborn slivers.

12 large eggs, preferably cage-free or omega-3, not too fresh (at least a week old)

1. Place the eggs in a Dutch oven or saucepan large enough to hold them snugly in a single layer. Cover the eggs with cool tap water.
2. Bring the water to a rolling boil over high heat; boil 1 minute. (Don't worry about the clatter in the pan.) Remove the saucepan from the heat; cover and let stand at room temperature 20 minutes.
3. Pour most of the hot water from the pan, leaving the eggs. Add cold tap water to the saucepan until overflowing and the hot water is rinsed out. Let stand in cool water 5 minutes before peeling the eggs you want immediately. Chill remainder, unpeeled, up to 1 week.

TIP: Use a smaller pan for cooking 6 eggs. The eggs should fit snugly in a single layer in the pan. Adding ice cubes to the cooling water can make shell removal even easier.

NUTRITIONAL INFORMATION PER SERVING
Calories: 155 • Protein: 13 g • Fat: 11 g • Carbohydrates: 1 g • Sugar: 1 g • Total fiber: 0 g • Sodium: 124 mg

THE ONLY GUACAMOLE RECIPE YOU'LL EVER NEED

Technique: Assemble
Tools: Chef's knife
Preparation time: 10 minutes
Servings: 4 (¼ cup each)

During two days alone, Super Bowl Sunday and Cinco de Mayo, Americans eat nearly 22 million pounds of guacamole. But there's no need to reserve it for special occasions; avocados are rich in heart-healthy monounsaturated fat and a good source of vitamins C and K. So, savor the guac. Just don't eat it straight from the serving bowl—or the chips right out of the bag.

Enjoy this simple, flavor-rich dip with fresh-cut vegetables or chips, and consider it as an alternative to ketchup, mayo, and butter. Spread it on a high-fiber low-carb tortilla and top it with leftover Roast Chicken (page 219), diced jalapeños or serranos, more cilantro, kosher salt, and freshly ground black pepper. Add diced red onion for color and crunch. It is delicious any time of day, for lunch or dinner, or even as part of a savory breakfast.

> 1 large ripe avocado, preferably Hass, peeled, seeded, and diced
> 3 tablespoons good-quality salsa, preferably hot or medium-hot, such as
>   Totally Natural Salpica Salsa
> ½ teaspoon garlic salt
> 2 tablespoons chopped fresh cilantro
> Vegetable dippers, such as carrot sticks, sliced peeled jicama, broccoli and
>   cauliflower florets
> Multigrain tortilla chips, such as Garden of Eatin'

1. Combine the avocado, salsa, and garlic salt in a medium bowl.
2. Use a fork to mash to desired consistency. Stir in or top with the cilantro.
3. Serve with vegetable dippers and/or tortilla chips.

TIP: The guacamole will last up to three days in the fridge. Sprinkle the surface with lemon or lime juice to prevent browning. In a pinch, press plastic wrap onto the guacamole surface to exclude air; because the guac is not heated, the plastic is okay.

SUBSTITUTIONS: Onion salt may replace the garlic salt and chopped green onion may replace the cilantro.

NUTRITIONAL INFORMATION PER SERVING (GUACAMOLE ONLY)
Calories: 64 • Protein: 1 g • Fat: 6 g • Carbohydrates: 4 g • Sugar: 1 g • Total fiber: 3 g • Sodium: 183 mg

SPICY TERIYAKI BROCCOLI

Technique: Stir-fry
Tools: Chef's knife, Dutch oven
Preparation time: 15 minutes
Cooking time: 7 minutes
Servings: 4 (²⁄₃ cup each)

Broccoli and stir-frying are a match made in cooking heaven. The high heat quickly cooks through the dense florets, transforming them from a dull hunter green to Technicolor emerald. If you prefer your broccoli al dente—tender crisp—you'll want to remove it from the heat when the veggie has just turned vividly bright. Even then, a knife should pierce the stem easily.

Dark sesame oil lends a pungent and nutty sheen of flavor. Made from roasted or toasted sesame seeds, this mahogany-hued oil is popular in Asian cuisine and is best for drizzling on a stir-fry just before serving. A little goes a long way, so drizzle gently, a drop at a time. Since you only use a small amount of this oil at a time, it's important to store properly. I suggest keeping it in the fridge, where it is dark and cool; make sure it is capped to prevent its becoming rancid from air exposure.

 4 cups small broccoli florets (cut from 1 large bunch broccoli or 10 ounces
    packaged fresh florets)
 4 garlic cloves, smashed, coarsely chopped
 2 tablespoons reduced-sodium soy sauce or tamari
 1 tablespoon dark sesame oil
 ½ teaspoon crushed red pepper flakes
 1 teaspoon toasted sesame seeds

1. Place the broccoli and garlic in a cold Dutch oven, stainless-steel skillet, or cast-iron skillet (do not use a nonstick skillet).
2. Combine the soy sauce, sesame oil, and red pepper flakes in a small bowl; mix well. Drizzle 1 tablespoon of the mixture over the broccoli in the skillet. Stir 2 tablespoons water into the remaining soy sauce mixture; set aside.

3. Turn the heat under the skillet to high. Stir-fry the mixture until hot and beginning to smoke, about 5 minutes. Turn off the heat, add the reserved soy sauce mixture, and stand back while the broccoli steams for 2 minutes. Toss well and serve topped with sesame seeds.

TIP: If using a head of broccoli, reserve the stems to chop for a stir-fry later in the week.

SUBSTITUTIONS: You can replace the soy sauce with 2 tablespoons of bottled teriyaki sauce (such as Soy Vey). The Soy Vey brand is a sweet liquid miracle and makes for an awesome marinade. It does have 5 grams of sugar per tablespoon, so don't drink it, even though you might be tempted.

Peanut or canola oil may replace the sesame oil, with some loss of flavor.

Spicy Brussels Sprouts: Exchange 1 pound of Brussels sprouts, trimmed and sliced through their cores into thin wedges, for the broccoli florets.

NUTRITIONAL INFORMATION PER SERVING
Calories: 60 • Protein: 3 g • Fat: 4 g • Carbohydrates: 5 g • Sugar: 0 g • Total fiber: 2 g • Sodium: 307 mg

CAULIFLOWER POPCORN

Technique: Roast
Tools: Chef's knife, rimmed baking sheet/jelly roll pan
Preparation time: 8 minutes
Cooking time: 18 minutes
Servings: 6 (about ¾ cup each)

Cauliflower experienced a renaissance a decade or so ago when foodies of the low-carb variety turned it into a mashed-potato substitute. Pureed with salt and pepper and a bit of cream, it makes for a satisfying vegetable side dish, but I think it is much tastier, more colorful, and more filling when roasted and dressed with some herbs and spices.

Roasting at high heat caramelizes the florets while maintaining their crispness. Resist the urge to speed up the cooking process with any temperature above 425 degrees—this will toast the outside of the cauliflower and leave the insides undercooked. You can enjoy this as a snack or serve it as a side dish. Turning the florets halfway through the cooking is nice, but not essential.

I head cauliflower, preferably organic, or 1½ pounds packaged cauliflower
    florets, or 6 cups florets from the salad bar
1½ tablespoons olive oil
½ teaspoon coarse sea salt or kosher salt
½ teaspoon freshly ground black pepper
¼ cup finely grated Parmigiano-Reggiano or aged Asiago cheese

1. Heat the oven to 425°F.
2. If using whole cauliflower, core the head, and cut into florets. Arrange florets on a 15-x-10-inch rimmed baking sheet. Drizzle the oil over the florets and sprinkle with salt and pepper. Toss well and spread in a single layer.
3. Bake 18 minutes or until golden brown on bottom. Transfer to a serving bowl; top with the cheese and toss.

Curried Cauliflower: Sprinkle ½ teaspoon curry powder or smoked paprika over the florets along with the salt and pepper.

Moroccan Cauliflower: Add ½ teaspoon ground cumin, ¼ teaspoon ground cinnamon, and ½ teaspoon ground coriander to the salt and pepper and sprinkle on the cauliflower.

NUTRITIONAL INFORMATION PER SERVING
Calories: 75 • Protein: 3 g • Fat: 5 g • Carbohydrates: 6 g • Sugar: 2 g • Total fiber: 2 g • Sodium: 245 mg

JAMAICAN TWO-BEAN VEGGIE SOUP

Technique: Simmer
Tools: Large saucepan or dutch oven, chef's knife
Preparation time: 5 minutes
Cooking time: 35 minutes
Servings: 8 (about I cup each)

Kale, peanut butter, and onion walk into a bar. The bartender says, "Not even Tom Cruise could make a cocktail with you three." Maybe not a cocktail, but a tasty island soup is Mission Possible.

Eight cups might seem like a lot of kale, but it cooks down significantly, and you should jump at any chance you get to bulk up on this superfood. Kale has been shown to cut the risk of certain types of cancer, such as bladder, colon, and prostate. High in sulfur, it can help stimulate the natural detoxification process that occurs in the liver.

If you are looking for a dense, flavorful, meat-free soup, this one, with its combination of unexpected flavors, is a showstopper. Jerk is a signature combination of spices, herbs, and condiments that make the Caribbean island marinades so unapologetically spicy and uniquely delicious. Jerk seasoning takes some time to make from scratch, and fortunately you can find it in dry and liquid forms at your local supermarket. If you don't already have it, it is a must for a Refuel pantry (#pantrycollection). You can use it in marinades for chicken or fish, and to spice up an oil-and-vinegar salad dressing. And sprinkling it on top of your hard-cooked or scrambled eggs will give your breakfast or snack a special kick.

I tablespoon olive oil

I medium onion, diced

2 tablespoons plus $1/2$ teaspoons jerk seasoning

I 32-ounce can vegetable broth, such as Imagine or Pacific

8 cups packed chopped kale leaves, from 2 bunches fresh kale, tough stems
    removed

I 15- or 16-ounce can no-salt-added black beans, rinsed and drained

I 16-ounce can no-salt-added red beans, rinsed and drained

I 14.5-ounce can diced tomatoes (organic preferred), with juice

I tablespoon natural peanut butter

1. Heat the oil in a large saucepan over medium heat. Add the onion and 2 tablespoons of the jerk seasoning; cook, stirring frequently, 5 minutes.

2. Add the remaining ingredients except the remaining jerk seasoning. Bring to a boil over high heat, reduce the heat, and simmer 25 to 30 minutes or until the vegetables are tender and the soup is slightly thickened.

3. Ladle the soup into shallow bowls; sprinkle ¼ teaspoon of the remaining seasoning over each serving.

TIPS: For a thicker soup, mash 1 cup of the red beans in a bowl before
stirring them into the soup. The leftover soup will keep up to 3 days in
the refrigerator or 3 months in the freezer.

SUBSTITUTIONS: Use 4 large shallots to replace the onion. Swiss chard may
replace the kale: chard is also beautiful, cruciferous, and a powerhouse
of nutrition. Kidney beans may replace the red beans.

NUTRITIONAL INFORMATION PER SERVING
Calories: 181 • Protein: 9 g • Fat: 3 g • Carbohydrates: 28 g • Sugar: 4 g • Total fiber: 7 g •
Sodium: 386 mg

PAN-SEARED MAHIMAHI
WITH RED CABBAGE

Technique: Sauté/stir-fry
Tools: Whisk, chef's knife, skillet
Preparation time: 10 minutes
Cooking time: 16 minutes
Servings: 2

Vermouth is the secret ingredient in this excellent fish dish. Technically
a fortified white wine flavored with dry ingredients (herbs, spices, fruits,
aromatics), vermouth has been sadly relegated to the back of the liquor
cabinet and has held long-distance-cousin status in cooking until very
recently. That's a shame because it has a range far beyond the classic
dry martini for which it is most famous. After all, it was herbal and medicinal before herbal and medicinal were hip.

Red cabbage is more than just a grunt ingredient in a coleslaw mix:
it's a dense, robust vegetable rich in fiber and also has excellent antioxidant and anti-inflammatory properties, displayed in its vibrant color,
a result of anthocyanin polyphenols. (Say that three times quickly, and
you get dinner.) When sautéed, red cabbage's moist ruffled interior can
turn velvety and steamy, a hearty vegetable side that you'll want to
make over and over again. If you're feeling continental, try the Italian

red cabbage (radicchio) variation and you'll get a contrasting, sophisti-
cated, slightly bitter layer of flavor.

> **4 teaspoons olive oil**
>
> **2 teaspoons Dijon mustard**
>
> **I tablespoon dry vermouth, dry sherry, dry white wine, or white wine vinegar**
>
> **2 4- to 5-ounce skinless mahimahi fillets**
>
> **4 I-inch-thick wedges red cabbage, cut through core from a small head (about 8 ounces)**
>
> **¼ teaspoon coarse sea salt or kosher salt**
>
> **¼ teaspoon freshly ground black pepper**
>
> **I tablespoon honey**
>
> **4 lemon wedges**

1. Whisk together 2 teaspoons of the oil and 1 teaspoon of the mustard; whisk in vermouth. Pour the mixture over the fish in a shallow
   plate or pie plate; set aside.
2. Drizzle the remaining 2 teaspoons oil over the cut sides of the cabbage wedges. Heat a large stainless-steel skillet over medium-high
   heat. Add the cabbage; cook 3 to 4 minutes per side or until browned
   and crisp-tender. Transfer to two serving plates; set aside.
3. Add the fish, with marinade still clinging, to the same skillet; cook
   over medium heat 3 to 4 minutes per side, or until opaque in center.
   Transfer to the serving plates; sprinkle the salt and pepper over.
4. Mix the honey and remaining 1 teaspoon mustard; drizzle over the
   cut sides of the cabbage. Serve with lemon wedges for squeezing
   over the fish.

SUBSTITUTIONS: Halibut may substitute for the mahimahi. Radicchio may
substitute for the cabbage.

NUTRITIONAL INFORMATION PER SERVING
Calories: 253 • Protein: 23 g • Fat: 10 g • Carbohydrates: 17 g • Sugar: 12 g • Total fiber: 3 g •
Sodium: 481 mg

ROAST CHICKEN WITH LEMON AND GARLIC JUICES

Technique: Roast
Tools: Chef's knife, roasting pan
Preparation time: 15 minutes
Cooking time: 55 to 60 minutes
Standing time: 15 minutes
Servings: 6

Many famous chefs say they would include a roast chicken in their imagined last supper. When chicken is well roasted, its tender, herb-infused succulence is addictive and appropriate for any occasion.

This roasted chicken recipe has few bells and whistles upfront, but there are fireworks of flavor at the end. The ratio of modest prep to the multisensory reward makes this a no-brainer. Best of all, you can't mess it up even if you try.

Preheat the oven as soon as you walk in the door. Change your clothes, prep the chicken, and slide it into the oven. Resist the urge to check frequently on the chicken as it roasts, as it will cause your oven to lose valuable heat. In about an hour, you'll have a supper that requires only a side dish or two to complete. Make this instead of picking up a supermarket rotisserie chicken, which can have over 1,500 milligrams of sodium in 6 ounces of meat.

  1 3- to 4-pound chicken, preferably organic
  4 thyme sprigs
  1 lemon, preferably organic, quartered
  4 garlic cloves, smashed
  1 tablespoon coarse sea salt or kosher salt
  $\frac{1}{2}$ teaspoon freshly ground black pepper

1. Heat the oven to 450°F. Rinse the chicken, then dry very well with paper towels, inside and out. Place the thyme sprigs, lemon, and garlic in the cavity. Tie the legs together with twine or a long twist tie. Place the chicken, breast side up, in a shallow roasting pan. Sprinkle the salt and pepper evenly over the chicken.

2. Roast the chicken for 55 to 60 minutes, or until the legs move easily in their sockets and the juices run clear (internal temperature of thigh should be 165°F).

3. Use a long-handled fork inserted into the cavity to tip the chicken so the juices run into the roasting pan; set pan aside. Transfer the chicken to a carving board with an indentation, or "tree" (or place the carving board into a rimmed baking sheet) to catch the juices. Let stand 15 minutes.

4. Carve the chicken into serving pieces. Combine the reserved pan juices and any juices from the carving board, and drizzle over the chicken. Discard the thyme, lemon, and garlic; save the carcass for making chicken stock, if desired.

TIP: Any leftover chicken may be refrigerated up to 3 days. Use to make Refuel Chicken Salad (page 221).

SUBSTITUTIONS: Rosemary, parsley, or oregano sprigs may replace the thyme sprigs.

NUTRITIONAL INFORMATION PER SERVING (WITHOUT SKIN)
Calories: 168 • Protein: 24 g • Fat: 7 g • Carbohydrates: 0 g • Sugar: 0 g • Total fiber: 0 g •
Sodium: 250 mg

⟩ ORGANIC MATTERS

When Korean researchers put a group of study participants on a five-day vegetarian program, their levels of endocrine disrupters and antibiotics significantly decreased. Here's what was cut out of their diet: industrially raised foods, such as beef, pork, and dairy, chock-full of hormone-disrupting chemicals and antibiotics.

You don't have to become a vegetarian to avoid antibiotics and endocrine disrupters, but you would be wise to buy organic, pasture-raised meats when possible. Certified organic farms must restrict the use of antibiotics in livestock, and the reduced use of pesticides also means fewer of these poisons will be passed on to you.

REFUEL CHICKEN SALAD

Technique: Assemble
Tools: Chef's knife
Preparation time: 15 minutes
Servings: 4 (about ½ cup each)

There are practically as many varieties of chicken salad as there are cooks. This one is lively and hearty, and should not be written off just because it has the word *salad* in the title—it's protein-focused instead of mayo-centered, and it pops with texture.

Even though we skip the gut-busting mayonnaise here, there's no sacrifice of creaminess and flavor. Toasted nuts transform this mix into a crunch-filled meal that can be enjoyed without the mandatory sandwich bread, which is better saved for a revival from hypoglycemia. Toast the nuts at 350 degrees for 5 minutes in a toaster oven or for about 7 minutes in a standard oven—you'll know they are done when they are fragrant. Once you master this recipe, try the tuna variation.

¼ cup low-fat sour cream
I tablespoon spicy brown mustard
2 cups chopped cooked chicken
¼ cup slivered almonds, toasted

1. In a medium bowl, mix the sour cream and mustard.
2. Stir in the chicken and almonds.
3. Serve over mixed greens or wrap in a low-carb, high-fiber tortilla.

TIP: Use any leftover meat from the Roast Chicken with Lemon and Garlic Juices (page 219) or from a store-bought rotisserie chicken.

SUBSTITUTIONS: Use your favorite kind of mustard in place of the spicy brown mustard. I love Grey Poupon. Pecans may replace the almonds.

Refuel Tuna Salad: Substitute a 12-ounce can of white tuna in water, drained, for the chicken; use 2 tablespoons finely chopped pickle (any kind) for the mustard; and ¼ cup chopped celery and 1 hard-cooked egg, peeled and chopped, for the almonds. (Calories: 138, protein: 21 g, fat: 4 g, carbs: 2 g, sugar: 2 g, total fiber: 0 g, sodium: 357 mg)

NUTRITIONAL INFORMATION PER SERVING
Calories: 199 • Protein: 22 g • Fat: 10 g • Carbohydrates: 2 g • Sugar: 1 g • Total fiber: 1 g • Sodium: 107 mg

GRILLED SIRLOIN STEAK AND ASPARAGUS

Technique: Grill
Tools: Tongs, chef's knife, carving board
Preparation time: 10 minutes
Cooking time: 14 minutes
Servings: 4

I'll let you in on a little secret about sirloin: grill it to the temperature the meat gods intended—medium rare—and you'll be rewarded with a tender, flavor-rich experience. Do not walk away from this fine-grained cut of meat, or it'll come back to haunt you. In a matter of 30 seconds, you can have an overcooked steak on your hands—one that's tough, dry, and drained of flavor. I use finger touch to monitor the grilling progress, but an instant-read thermometer and the touch of tongs work well (revisit the Tongs & Touch Test on page 189).

To get a bigger, bolder rosemary flavor (think pine cone meets fire), use fresh rosemary instead of dried. Remove the green, spiky leaves from the stem and chop finely. The standard rule for herb and spice equivalents is that you need three times as much fresh herb as you do dried. But rosemary is especially pungent even when fresh, so I would stick with 2 teaspoons fresh to start.

Prep the asparagus by bending each spear near the bottom until it breaks naturally; or, if you want to guess how much is tender and how much is not, slice off the bottom 1½ inches. Toss out the tougher end pieces. Grilling the asparagus brings out the best in this spring vegetable; done to the right crispness, you'll wish you had more than one bunch.

2 tablespoons olive oil
2 teaspoons dried rosemary leaves, crushed with fingers

1 1-pound boneless top sirloin steak about 1 inch thick, preferably grass fed

1 tablespoon balsamic vinegar

1 bunch (1 to 1¼ pounds) fresh asparagus spears, ends trimmed

½ teaspoon coarse sea salt or kosher salt

½ teaspoon freshly ground black pepper

2 tablespoons finely grated Parmigiano-Reggiano or Asiago cheese

1. Use a paper towel with a little olive oil or olive oil cooking spray to coat a cold, clean grill. Then, heat gas grill to medium or prepare charcoals, letting the coals burn until they are covered with a gray ash and are medium-hot.

2. Press the rosemary onto both sides of the steak. Mix 1 tablespoon of the oil with the vinegar in a shallow plate or pie plate. Add the steak, turning to coat, and press in any rosemary that fell away from the meat.

3. Place the asparagus in another shallow plate. Drizzle the remaining 1 tablespoon oil over the asparagus, turning to coat lightly.

4. Grill the steak (with marinade clinging), covered, over medium-high heat 3 to 4 minutes per side, for medium-rare. Transfer the steak to a carving board; tent with foil and let stand 10 minutes.

5. Meanwhile, grill the asparagus until crisp-tender, 4 to 5 minutes, rolling asparagus with tongs occasionally. Transfer to four serving plates.

6. Carve the steak across the grain into thin slices; transfer to the plates with the asparagus. Sprinkle the salt and pepper over the steak and asparagus; sprinkle the cheese over the asparagus. Drizzle any juices from the carving board over the steak.

TIP: Save any leftovers (steak already thinly sliced) for wrapping in a high-fiber, low-carb tortilla with chopped lettuce or vegetables, perfect for a grab-and-go lunch.

NUTRITIONAL INFORMATION PER SERVING
Calories: 254 • Protein: 29 g • Fat: 13 g • Carbohydrates: 5 g • Sugar: 2 g • Total fiber: 2 g •
Sodium: 336 mg

REFUEL BEEF STEW

Technique: Simmer
Tools: Large saucepan or Dutch oven, chef's knife
Preparation time: 10 minutes
Cooking time: 1 hour
Servings: 4 (1¼ cups each)

Classic winter comfort food (check). Hearty, warm, and satisfying (check). You can't stop eating it (check). Hunters and gatherers from times long ago wanted the rich, deep flavor of beef stew, with great gravy. And the good news for today's men is that it's relatively inexpensive, filling, and, after you've done it a few times, intuitive.

My version is perfect for a weekend, when you can give it an hour's cooking time. You're rewarded with an inside track to several chef's tricks: sear to create a crust; add a flavorful broth (not water); use a good red wine (I like Syrah, Merlot, Cabernet Sauvignon, and Cabernet Franc); and cook the mushrooms down to build layers of flavor. Then it's simmer time. If you're ambitious—or hungry—triple this recipe.

You can expect family members or guests to wander into the kitchen for a bite of goodness. Leftovers are hard to come by with this meal, but they are delicious. When you reheat the stew, add a bit of broth first.

I pound boneless beef chuck (in 1-inch pieces), preferably grass fed
2 tablespoons whole wheat flour
1 tablespoon dried thyme
1 tablespoon olive oil
6 garlic cloves, smashed, then coarsely chopped
2 8-ounce packages sliced button mushrooms
1½ cups reduced-sodium beef broth, such as Imagine or Pacific
1 cup dry red wine
1 14.5-ounce can diced tomatoes, with juice
2 tablespoons Worcestershire sauce
¼ cup chopped Italian parsley (optional)

1. Toss the meat with the flour and thyme. Heat the oil in a large saucepan or Dutch oven over medium-high heat. Add the meat; cook 3 minutes, stirring once.
2. Add the garlic and cook 1 to 2 minutes, until fragrant, stirring once. Add the mushrooms and cook 3 minutes, stirring once. Add the broth, wine, tomatoes, and Worcestershire sauce; bring to a boil, stirring once.
3. Reduce the heat to medium and simmer, uncovered, 55 minutes or until the meat is fork-tender, stirring once. Ladle into shallow bowls; garnish with parsley, if desired.

SUBSTITUTIONS: Dried oregano leaves may replace the thyme leaves, cremini (baby bella) mushrooms may replace the button mushrooms, and additional beef broth may replace the red wine.

NUTRITIONAL INFORMATION PER SERVING
Calories: 303 • Protein: 28 g • Fat: 9 g • Carbohydrates: 18 g • Sugar: 7 g • Total fiber: 2 g • Sodium: 608 mg

EASY HOMEMADE BREAKFAST SAUSAGE

Technique: Sauté/stir-fry
Tools: Box grater, stainless-steel skillet
Preparation time: 10 minutes
Cooking time: 8 to 10 minutes
Servings: 4 (2 patties each)

Just about every country has its version of sausage—you'll find bangers in Britain, bratwurst in Germany, and kielbasa in Poland. One trait these variations on ground processed meat share is that they are often cooked at high temperatures or charred. Meats so tortured have been linked to pancreatic, lung, and colon cancer. The nasty chemicals generated with high-heat meat cooking also happen to be estrogenic.

You can cut out the preservatives and extra calories by making your own version of sausage with ground turkey, and cooking it gently. The flesh of the apple melts into the turkey while the apple skin gives it a firmer chew, like you're truly eating something. The poultry seasoning allows you to lower the fat without sacrificing flavor. A whiff from the jar may take you on a quick trip to Thanksgiving Day—this blend of thyme, sage, marjoram, rosemary, black pepper, and nutmeg is often added to the traditional holiday stuffing.

I pound 93% fat-free ground turkey
I large egg
$\frac{1}{2}$ cup grated unpeeled apple, preferably organic
$1\frac{1}{2}$ teaspoons poultry seasoning
I teaspoon onion salt
$\frac{1}{2}$ teaspoon freshly ground black pepper

1. In a medium bowl, mix all the ingredients with your hands. Form into 8 patties about ½ inch thick and 3 inches in diameter.
2. Heat in a large stainless-steel skillet coated with olive oil cooking spray and add the patties. Cook over medium-low heat 4 to 5 minutes on each side, or until no longer pink in the center. Remove and serve.

SUBSTITUTIONS: Ground sage may replace poultry seasoning. Garlic salt may replace onion salt.

NUTRITIONAL INFORMATION PER SERVING
Calories: 178 • Protein: 24 g • Fat: 8 g • Carbohydrates: 3 g • Sugar: I g • Total fiber: I g • Sodium: 267 mg

Seafood Sausage. Substitute 1 can (3 ounces) smoked oysters, drained and finely chopped, or drained and chopped smoked herring (kippers), for the apple. (Calories: 216, protein: 28 g, fat: 11 g, carbs: 4 g, sugar: 0 g, total fiber: 2 g, sodium: 364 mg)

TIP: For a quick lunch, wrap two patties in aluminum foil. Put them and two hard-cooked eggs and an apple in your bag, and you're set.

> ## THE FIFTH FLAVOR
> Oysters bring the flavor of umami to a dish. The term *umami* is Japanese and means "pleasant, savory, and delicious" all rolled into one satisfying bite. It's not fishy, but is rich and salty, giving dishes including the breakfast sausage a deep, dense layer of flavor.

CENTRAL MEXICAN CHILI

Technique: Simmer
Tools: Large saucepan, chef's knife
Preparation time: 5 minutes
Cooking time: 20 minutes
Servings: 5 (I cup each)

I was privileged to cook in Rick Bayless's famed Chicago restaurant, Topolobampo, which spurred my own passion for Mexican food, with its amazing flavors. I could eat Mexican food every day. Sometimes I do.

Central Mexican food pulls in influences from all around Mexico, but here I use its quality of restraint—no heavy-handed piles of cheese, beans, or meat, but just enough of each, suffused with chilies and fresh herbs. Look for a chili powder that has no salt or chemical additives, and consider it often in cooking—it can be added to whatever ground or shredded meat you have on hand.

This chili always works and always tastes great. Don't skip the toppings—they add texture, color, and cooling goodness.

I pound 93% fat-free ground turkey
I tablespoon salt-free chili powder, preferably Spice Hunter or Gebhardt's
I 14.5-ounce can diced tomatoes (organic preferred), with juice
I cup all-natural salsa, preferably hot or medium
I 16-ounce can no-salt-added kidney beans, drained (no need to rinse)
I ripe medium avocado, preferably Hass, peeled, seeded, and diced
5 tablespoons low-fat sour cream
½ cup chopped cilantro

1. Cook the turkey in a large saucepan over medium heat, stirring frequently, 5 minutes or until no longer pink. Stir in the chili powder and cook 1 minute more.
2. Stir in the tomatoes, salsa, and beans; simmer uncovered 15 minutes, or until slightly thickened, stirring occasionally.
3. Ladle chili into shallow bowls; top with avocado, sour cream, and cilantro.

TIPS: For a subtle sweetness, add ¼ teaspoon ground cinnamon along with the chili powder. Leftover chili may be refrigerated up to 3 days or frozen up to 3 months.

SUBSTITUTIONS: Pinto beans may replace the kidney beans and green onions may replace the cilantro. Lean ground beef, preferably grass fed, can replace the turkey.

NUTRITIONAL INFORMATION PER SERVING
Calories: 296 • Protein: 25 g • Fat: 12 g • Carbohydrates: 25 g • Sugar: 5 g • Total fiber: 9 g • Sodium: 480 mg

COCONUT RICE PUDDING WITH BOURBON AND TOASTED PECANS

Technique: Simmer
Tools: Saucepan, chef's knife
Preparation time: 5 minutes
Cooking time: 15 minutes
Servings: 4 (²⁄₃ cup each)

Creamy coconut pudding always scores high on the pleasure scale. Is it the bourbon? The toasted pecans? The coconut milk? Nah; it's just that it's a dessert, and when you decide to have one, you've got to make sure that it's not the last one of the night. Make this smooth, light treat for your significant other on a cold night to enjoy by the fire, and you'll thank me later.

If you've never used stevia, touch a tiny sample to your tongue—it's up to 300 times sweeter than cane or beet sugar, so a little goes a long way. Two packets are enough to bring up the sweetness in this dollop of dessert without making it cloying. Who knows? If you're using Maker's Mark, you might not need stevia at all.

1 14-ounce can light unsweetened coconut milk
¾ cup unsweetened vanilla almond milk
¼ cup cornstarch
¾ cup cooked brown rice

2 packets pure stevia sweetener, such as Pyure or Truvia
1½ tablespoons good bourbon
¼ cup coarsely chopped pecans, toasted (see Tip)

1. Place the coconut milk in a medium saucepan. Stir ¼ cup of the almond milk into the cornstarch in a small bowl, stirring until cornstarch is completely dissolved. Add to the coconut milk along with the remaining almond milk and the rice, stirring well. Slowly bring to a simmer over medium heat, stirring frequently. Simmer, stirring frequently, until the mixture thickens, about 3 minutes.
2. Remove from the heat; stir in the stevia. Let stand uncovered in the saucepan 10 minutes, stirring once.
3. Stir in the bourbon; transfer to four old-fashioned glasses and top with the pecans. Serve warm, at room temperature, or chill for up to 3 days before serving.

TIP: Toast the nuts in the oven or a toaster oven at 350 degrees for 5 to 8 minutes, or until fragrant. You can toast 1 cup of nuts at one time and freeze the cooled extra nuts in a heavy plastic freezer bag for up to six months. It is a good idea to always mark a date on the outside of frozen items.

SUBSTITUTIONS: Erythritol, available as ZSweet, can be used instead of stevia. A good scotch whisky may replace the bourbon, and walnuts may replace the pecans.

NUTRITIONAL INFORMATION PER SERVING
Calories: 175 • Protein: 2 g • Fat: 9 g • Carbohydrates: 18 g • Sugar: 0 g • Total fiber: 2 g • Sodium: 45 mg

▶ BETTER THAN DESSERT

If you order dessert at a restaurant, you may as well skip having sex that night. The dessert weighs you down, and takes the oomph out of lovemaking. My advice is to skip the one that causes cavities, and indulge the one that, uh, doesn't. This works, of course, every time you think of having dessert, especially at night. In other words, dinner dates out don't have to finish with dessert at the restaurant; instead, reserve the sweet finale for when you get home.

REFUEL OFF-THE-SHELF MEALS AND SNACKS

In a time crunch for a meal or a snack? You can do better than a PB&J or the dollar menu. Use these ideas for snacks and dishes that require nothing more than a bit of assembly (some assume that you're using leftovers). They're simple, flavorful, and easy. Don't stress about the precise amounts of each ingredient—these edibles are made to be flexible.

Meals

1. Heat a can of vegetable soup (a few options: Healthy Choice, Eden Organic, or Trader Joe's) and top with quartered Babybel cheeses and fresh parsley. If the soup seems bland, stir in a little chili-garlic puree or salsa.

2. Spread whole corn tortillas or sturdy tostadas with natural peanut butter and sliced fresh strawberries or apple slices, a few sunflower seeds, and a sprinkle of ground cinnamon.

3. Purchase grilled vegetables from the deli and top with chunks of smoked trout and toasted slivered almonds.

4. Scramble some eggs with chopped onion and top with strips of smoked salmon.

5. Cook packaged pre-rinsed quinoa and stir in thawed frozen edamame or lima beans and halved pitted green or kalamata olives and a dash of the brine from the jar.

6. Grill or broil a meaty portobello mushroom brushed with Worcestershire sauce and sprinkled with Jamaican jerk or Cajun seasoning.

7. Steam mussels in white wine 5 minutes until opened and serve in a bowl with a drizzle of warmed lite coconut milk spiked with crushed red pepper flakes.

8. Split and seed a small butternut or acorn squash and roast cut-side-down until tender, then fill hollows with toasted pumpkin or squash seeds and a sprinkle of sea salt.

9. Toss packaged fresh coleslaw mix (cabbage and carrot) with a little soy sauce or teriyaki sauce, rice wine vinegar, and sesame oil. Stir in cilantro or green onion, if you have any.

10. Grill halibut or cod fillets and serve them in warm corn tortillas with salsa and diced avocado.

Snacks

1. Spread sliced roasted turkey breast with grainy mustard, top with sliced almonds, and roll up in a lettuce leaf.
2. Drain canned tuna in oil, add tomato salsa and coriander seeds to taste.
3. Drain a can of smoked oysters or kippers and serve on Terra vegetable chips instead of crackers.
4. Top hard-cooked egg halves with a spoonful of guacamole and a sprinkling of cumin seeds.
5. Mix shelled pistachios, mini chocolate chips, a little high-protein dry cereal, and a dash of cinnamon.

15

A FEAST ON THE RUN

How to Get the Most out of Meals Away from Home

Here's the truth: restaurants are not in the business of helping you lose your gut. If losing your gut is your goal, eating foods cooked or assembled in your own home or with your own hands, or the hands of someone who respects your goals, should become a priority.

However, the reality is that you are busy and the demands of your daily life are not going away anytime soon. This means that whatever your best intentions may be, you may get stuck flipping through a restaurant menu during a business meeting or at your kid's favorite diner. Or, you'll be at the newest local sushi spot for dinner with your wife, significant other, or friends. You might even be distracted by food porn on display at the drive-thru (see When Fast Food Is the Only Option, page 245). Do you panic and order what you always do? A man with a plan doesn't.

HOW TO GET GOOD AT GOING TO RESTAURANTS

These are dangerous, confusing times for the hungry man on the go. There are 1,800-calorie salads on the market, omelets with 82 grams of fat, sandwiches in which the bread has been replaced by pieces of fried chicken, and restaurants bearing the name "factory" (because nothing sounds better than a manufactured meal) that churn out diabetes-inducing portions fit for three. Sure, some of these items do nothing to hide their gut-bomb status, but others are a bit more stealthy.

One of the best ways to ensure you know what you're really eating is to look up nutritional info ahead of time and even pick out what you're going to order. Many people don't know that most restaurants, especially chain restaurants, have more nutritional info on hand than calories alone.

But I believe that you're the restaurant CEO when you dine out: ask for it, nicely, and they'll help you find it. Read on to learn how to order safely.

WALK ON BY

Impromptu meals don't leave you time to read *Yelp* reviews or search online for a place to eat (also impossible if you're in an area without cell service). Need to hit the sidewalk and search for a suitable place to dine? A few things should tell you to keep walking:

- Baskets of fluffy bread permanently on the tables
- No tables
- Tables or counters but no chairs
- Eye-catching neon signage and chairs—designed to get you in, fatten you up with cheap, sugary, fatty fast food, and get you out

If you have a laptop or smartphone with service, check out www.healthyout .com. Put in an address and then sort restaurants by calories, lowest carbs, or highest protein categories. Warning: your mileage and the nutritional quality may vary. But it's a start.

I'm going to arm you with some specific strategies for dish selections, but first, here are some tips to help you stay on track at any time.

Top 11 Strategies for Restaurant Survival :

I. **Send back the bread, chips, or other bottomless item offered upon being seated.** (Exception: relish trays, small dishes of pickled peppers, fresh radishes, jardinera. Bring 'em on.) Before you send an item back, however, offer it to your dining mates. These high-calorie, low-nutrient foods fill up valuable real estate in your stomach that should be reserved for foods that work for you, not poison you. Do you feel hungry or just have a reflex to eat when you sit down? Either way, order water with lemon for the table and drink yours first thing. Then ask for another glass. Take this time to catch up with your dining mates.

2. **Request a carryout container before you start.** Standard portions have ballooned beyond reasonable, so be proactive here. When you order, ask for a to-go box to come with your meal. Or, before it gets to you, try asking your server: "Could you put half of that in a takeout container for me?" Remember, if the food's there, you'll usually eat it (we're wired that way), so simply thinking you'll just eat half usually won't work. Divide your meal in half and stow the container under your chair while eating. Note to self: this is an option even for business meals and dates. Don't make a fuss of it; just respect the purpose of being together, which isn't to eat or drink, but to do business, socialize, or romance. If you're in a fine-dining restaurant, there's a decent chance you won't get a portion of meat or fish that's larger than a deck of cards—in such cases, halving isn't necessary.

3. **Order according to the Five Refuel Commandments.** In restaurants serving American food, order undisguised lean fish, chicken, or tofu, grilled, broiled, or baked (that's your standing order), and substitute steamed or roasted vegetables for any grain, bun, or deep-fried or mashed side. Say, "I'll have the grilled fish of the day with light oil, no breading or coating, sauce on the side, double steamed vegetables instead of the starch."

4. **Request all sauces on the side, or replace them with lemon or Tabasco, salsa, or other hot sauce.** You can get a grilled piece of fish or chicken with vegetables or a salad at just about any diner or café. Save your splurge for a special meal: your birthday (not your cousin's), your anniversary (not the neighbors'), your job promotions (never count the money until it's in your account). TGIF doesn't count.

5. **Be politely precise and remember who's paying the check.** The wait staff is your connection to the chef. Make sure she or he knows what you want. When your meal comes, check it out—did you get what you ordered? If not, send it back. All of it. Reward attentive, careful service with a generous tip (20 percent or more). Be prepared to be in charge.

6. **Taste sauce before putting it on.** Saturated fats aren't the villain they were made

out to be in the eighties, but they do have 9 calories per gram (compared to carbohydrates and proteins, which have 4) and can add up quickly—especially with sauces. Taste is real: if it is rich or salty, you can tell by tasting. Dip your fork in the dressing. Don't pour it on your salad, especially unless you've tasted it. If your fork stands up in the dressing, the dressing will floor you with its calories and fat. Ask for lemon or rice wine vinegar and extra virgin olive oil instead.

7. **Eat the vegetables first.** Vegetables such as broccoli, cauliflower, or even a green salad should mark the official start of your meal. Full of nutrients and fiber, they will set the foundation for a satisfying experience.

8. **Pour coffee or salt on the food still in front of you if you don't want to be tempted to continue to eat. Or box it.** Sounds strange, but Refueled men have applied these strategies and they work. Restaurant food is salty to start with, and if you dump several shakes of salt onto the remains of your meal, you'll get a taste you'll never forget or want to repeat. Coffee, of course, will quickly put an end to picking. If you don't want to waste food, box half of it before your "I am full" notifier breaks down again, and put it out of sight, under your chair.

9. **Give the box to a homeless person on the way out.** If you don't need it, give it to someone who does.

10. **Drink water, especially if you have wine, before, during, and after a meal.** Any type of alcohol can minimize production of vasopressin, the antidiuretic hormone that regulates water retention and keeps your body hydrated. To counter this effect, drink water before, during, and after alcohol consumption. You'll prevent headache-inducing dehydration and flush your cells and tissues so they're not steeped in alcohol. And you'll keep your blood alcohol level down, and below DUI levels. Hydrate with at least 16 ounces of water for every 5-ounce glass of wine. And wait an hour before you decide to have another glass of wine.

11. **Skip dessert.** Early civilizations ate fruit and nuts for dessert; some modern ones still do. If you want something sweet to close a meal, you'd be wise to follow their lead instead of diving into a lava cake. The molten version offered by the Chili's chain will blast your belly out to volcanic proportions: 166 grams of carbs (they don't reveal how many of these are sugar, but I'd guess 165), 74 grams of fat, and a whopping 1,430 calories. Per serving. Generally, you should opt out of dessert, but in a restaurant, a sample of cheeses is the best option if you have to have something—the rich flavors and bit of fat will force you to eat slowly and enjoy, and also, cut the risk of pre-sleep snacking. Just be sure to track the calories. An ounce of cheese (about the size of your thumb) is 110+ calories. And remember what I said about having dessert twice in a night: it's unlikely.

> **MAN MEMO**
>
> Pasta dishes are often marked up nearly 1,000 percent: pasta is a cheap ingre-
> dient and pasta dishes are cheap to make. Unless you're in an Italian country-
> side café and waiters are greeting you with "*Buona sera, signore*" or it's a special
> occasion, you should opt for something other than a bowl of (probably over- or
> undercooked) pasta.

The Menu Decoder

There are more foods on menus that will dent your testosterone and
balloon your belly than there are those that won't. This is true no matter how much money you're spending on a meal out; even fine dining
doesn't equal a flat belly.

It helps to become familiar with the language of menus since
they're often written in food code, with some terms and phrases easier
to call out than others. Items can be especially hard to decipher when
they're written in an unfamiliar language, as is the case with most foreign languages. Ready yourself to make the right choices by studying
this Refuel Menu Decoder. You'll see which options you should avoid
(foul territory) and which you should choose (fair game).

THE REFUEL MENU DECODER	
FRENCH	
On the Menu	**Decoded**
Foul Territory	
Au gratin	Baked dish topped with breadcrumbs and grated cheese
Béchamel, béarnaise, and hollandaise sauces	Entrée sauces that accompany prepared meats and vegetables; these are made with heavy cream and butter
Fondue	Hot dish of melted cheese, into which bread cubes are dipped; also can be hot oil into which strips of meat are dipped
Pommes frites	French-fried potatoes

THE REFUEL MENU DECODER (continued)

Confit	Goose or duck, cooked and preserved in its own fat
Brioche, éclairs, croissants	Pastries made with a lot of butter

FRENCH

On the Menu	Decoded
Fair Game	
Salade Niçoise	Green salad with tuna (canned or seared), hard-cooked eggs, olives, and tomatoes
En papillote	Aromatic preparation, often of fish or chicken, that is wrapped in parchment and steamed
Steamed mussels	Mussels prepared in a broth of white wine, garlic, butter, and herbs; skip "frites," if they are part of the dish
Pot-au-feu	Boiled beef dish prepared with stock, wine, and herbs; broth is served first, then meat is sliced and served as entrée
Coulis	Fresh sauce of pureed vegetable or fruits, served with meats or fish
Nouvelle	"New cuisine"—*nouvelle* suggests lighter dishes

ITALIAN

Foul Territory	
Alfredo	Pasta sauce made with cream, butter, and cheese
Fritto or fritto misto	Mixed fried plate, usually seafood, eggplant, zucchini, or mozzarella sticks
Carbonara	Pasta sauce made with bacon, cream, eggs, and cheese
Parmigiano, parmigiana	Breaded and sautéed preparation of veal, chicken, or eggplant, served with a tomato sauce; can be baked instead, but not common in restaurants
Tortellini, ravioli, cannelloni, manicotti	Cheese- or meat-filled pastas
Cannoli	Fried thin pastry filled with sweetened ricotta

On the Menu	Decoded
THE REFUEL MENU DECODER (continued)	
Fair Game	
Antipasto	Dish of cured meats, cheeses, olives, and vegetables; means "pre-meal," but can be an entrée; choose vegetable antipasto if possible
Insalata caprese	Layered slices of fresh basil, tomato, and mozzarella, drizzled with olive oil
Minestrone	Thick soup of vegetables and beans
Cacciatore	Stew of meat, chicken, or rabbit, with tomatoes, onions, and herbs
Bistecca alla fiorentina	Broiled or grilled steak, seasoned with olive oil and lemon; definitely take half to go
Carpaccio	Thin slices of raw meat or fish, served as appetizer with olive oil, capers, fresh greens
CHINESE	
Foul Territory	
Crispy	Applied to anything deep-fried
Egg foo yung	Dish of eggs with vegetables and meat or shrimp, fried and then served with gravy
Lo mein	Chinese egg noodles cooked with vegetables and meat or shrimp and tossed in sauce
Chow mein	Chinese-American dish of fried noodles topped with stir-fried vegetables
Steamed or fried white rice	Steamed rice is served as accompaniment; fried rice is often part of an entrée; both are refined carbs, bad regardless of preparation
Won-tons	Filled dumplings, sometimes steamed and sometimes fried, served in soup or as appetizer
General Tso's chicken	Breaded and fried chicken dish, served with a syrupy sauce

THE REFUEL MENU DECODER (continued)

CHINESE

On the Menu	Decoded
Fair Game	
Spring rolls	Fresh (not fried) rice-paper rolls filled with vegetables
Szechuan	Spicy regional food style flavored with garlic and chilies
Kung pao	Chicken stir-fry dish, with chilies and peanuts
Hoisin, hot mustard, or oyster sauce	Condiments/ingredients for Chinese food, offering great flavor in small amounts
Moo goo gai pan	Stir-fried chicken and vegetables in a light sauce

JAPANESE

Foul Territory	
Agemono, tempura	Breaded and fried foods, typically shrimp or vegetables
Katsu	Chicken or pork cutlet, often fried
Fugu	Relative of pufferfish, dangerous if not prepared properly; try it only at an authentic Japanese sushi restaurant
Crunchy roll	Tempura-fried roll filled with fried ingredients
Ramen, udon, soba	Noodles, served in soups and also as entrées
Fair Game	
Sashimi	Slices of raw fish served with condiments such as wasabi and pickled ginger
Edamame	Boiled fresh soybeans, served as a vegetable
Pickled ginger	Thin slices of preserved ginger, served as a condiment with sushi and sashimi
Shabu-shabu	Fondue-style meal of meats and veggies, cooked in hot broth by the diner

THE REFUEL MENU DECODER (continued)

Negamaki	Pork or beef slices rolled around green onions, broiled and served with soy sauce

THAI/SOUTHEAST ASIAN

On the Menu	Decoded
Foul Territory	
Crab Rangoon	Burmese appetizer of crab and cheese-filled fried dumplings
Kao pad	Thai-style fried rice
Sticky (glutinous) rice	Short- or medium-grain rice, slightly sweet; ask for brown rice instead
Mi krop or mee krob	Crispy fried rice noodles, usually served with a sauce
Pad Thai	Thai stir-fried rice noodles with shrimp, peanuts, vegetables, and chilies; mostly carbs, sugar, and usually only a small amount of protein
Fair Game	
Gaeng pah (jungle curry)	Thai broth-based curry; can be spicy without the fat from coconut milk to cut the heat
Satay	Marinated cubes of meat, fish, or chicken on skewer and grilled, served with spicy peanut sauce
Larb	Laos/Thai grilled ground meats flavored with lime, fish sauce, and chilies
Red or green curry	Wide variety of spicy Asian stewlike dishes
Lemongrass	Flavorful grass used to flavor sauces with a citrus note

MEXICAN

Foul Territory	
Tortilla chips	Fried pieces of corn or flour tortillas
Nachos	Cheese-drizzled corn chips; goes straight to the gut

THE REFUEL MENU DECODER (continued)	
Taco salad	Green salad served in a large deep-fried tortilla-like bowl
Chalupas, chimichangas, tostadas	Dishes based on fried tortillas with minimal filling or topping
Chiles rellenos	Cheese-stuffed chilies, battered and deep-fried
Churros	Fried doughnuts sprinkled with cinnamon and sugar
Fair Game	
Arroz con pollo	Chicken and rice dish; replace the rice with black beans
Gazpacho	Cold tomato-cucumber soup
Ceviche	Raw fish that's been marinated in citrus juices, often with onion, tomato, spices, and cilantro
Fajitas	Grilled strips of meat or seafood served in a flour tortilla; replace with a corn tortilla
Taco al carbon or al pastor	Grilled marinated meats served in a soft corn tortilla
Fish taco	Grilled fish and cabbage, served in a soft corn tortilla; ask for no white sauce, and add a squeeze of lemon and some hot sauce

THE TRAVELIN' MAN

Being a road warrior might move you up the corporate ladder, but it will also pack on the pounds, increase your stress and blood pressure, and lead to sleep disturbances. Many of my patients travel too much, and they have 40 extra pounds to show for it.

But those pounds don't have to be a permanent side effect of your business travel. You can learn how to eat right on the go. You do have to plan, and you do have to invest a little time. But you can do that strategically, and it will save your waistline, your heart, and your gonads.

To avoid travel pitfalls, use the Five Refuel Commandments (page 103). The top three to keep in mind are: Don't eat foods you can crush, Look for undisguised proteins and strong vegetables, and Drink plenty of citrus water (plain water works, too, when you can't track down fruit). Respect the rules, and you'll survive. Because it's a jungle out there.

Here are other some rules for when you hit the road or take to the sky, whether for business or pleasure:

On a Plane

- **Eat before you go.** This might seem like an obvious tip, but not if your typical plan involves eating at the airport while you wait for your flight. Eat at home, where you'll maintain complete control of what you're eating.
- **Air travel is designed for traveling, not for eating.** Basically, jets are to get you from one place to another. You're captive, and people now expect that being captive means you'll be fed. It's reflexive. But you don't have to eat, especially if you are not hungry. You do have to drink water, because plane air is dehydrating. If you do eat, bring your own food. (#BYOF)
- **Bring your water bottle and skip sodas and alcohol on the plane.** Dehydration will lead to fatigue, irritability, headaches, and constipation. Bring an empty stainless-steel or BPA-free bottle. Once you're through security, ask at a bar or coffee shop to fill the bottle with water. On the plane, drink water or soda water with lime or lemon.
- **Stuck in the airport? Go Mexican.** Guacamole and salsa with carne asada or pollo asado are great restaurant choices; beans and rice are less ideal, but still substantially better than the chili cheese fries and giganti-burger available a few gates down.

▶ WOULD YOU LIKE A WINDOW OR AN AISLE SEAT, SIR?

There are worse things on a plane than a wayward elbow or a scream-happy toddler—there are blood clots. Called deep venous thrombosis, blood clots lodged in your leg can cause painful swelling, thrombophlebitis, or in the worst case, pulmonary embolism. While the overall risk is minor, being overweight or obese increases your chances of developing blood clots. Researchers from the American College of Chest Physicians found that sitting in a window seat also significantly increases the risk of blood clots, as you're a lot more likely to stay put. Select an aisle seat, stretch your calves, and take the short walk to the bathroom to improve your circulation.

On the Road

PACK YOUR OWN FOOD When you have time to prepare for a road trip, your cooler should be just as much a priority as your luggage. Pack chicken or fish or steak leftovers without dressing so they don't get soggy, toss in a few small apples and some almonds or pistachios in the shell, and as many hard-cooked eggs as you can fit, as well as plenty of water, with an extra lemon or lime. Long stretches of highway offer ample time for mindless snacking. To curb this habit, chew xylitol-sweetened sugarless gum (it helps to fight cavities and you don't get enough xylitol to cause diarrhea), and reach for your citrus water instead. When genuine hunger hits, snack on Refuel Trail Mix (page 206) instead of fiery hot crispy chips or other such crap.

GRAB THIS AT THE GAS STATION If you didn't bring your own food, and hunger hits at the quickie mart or gas station snack shop, pass by the candy and protein bar (aka candy) rack. Go for perishable goods in the refrigerated section: low-sugar yogurt and cheese sticks are good; hard-cooked eggs are a lot better (most 7–Elevens carry them). Elsewhere in the store, look for your new old standbys: unsweetened beef, turkey, or salmon jerky; nuts; and small bags of trail mix, preferably without chocolate, raisins, and pretzels.

DINERS AND THE DOUBLE D I love Guy Fieri's *Diners, Drive-Ins, and Dives,* on the Food Network. But he left off the other double D: Die and Dying.

Restaurants like those are actually better choices than fast-food joints, and the people running diners and dives are often great cooks, but you've got to be careful. They're eateries of, umm, special occasion. Soups and salads are often a safe choice, if you ask for the salad with everything on the side, and vegetables to crunch instead of crackers. For breakfast, an omelet stuffed with veggies, light on the cheese and butter, can be a smart choice. Excessive use of both is pretty much guaranteed at a diner.

Other options are cottage cheese with tomatoes, hard-cooked or other prepared eggs, or a nice strong cup of coffee. Don't loiter to pick at your companion's fries or hash browns or toast, or tiny packets of jam laden with high-fructose corn syrup or something else you don't really want—you've got places to go.

GO THE EXTRA HALF MILE If you get off the highway just a bit more, you can typically find a local grocery store. Do this before you check into a hotel, too—it's way smarter (and cheaper) than room service. Step inside that decent-size supermarket and grab the pull-tab cans of tuna or salmon (pouches work, too), a lemon or an orange, and a bag of prewashed lettuce. Look for salt and pepper packets and utensils on the way out. If the store has a salad bar, you can also use the Refuel Rules for Navigating the Salad Bar:

1. Walk all the way around so you see everything.
2. Go back to the beginning and get the size container that you want to eat now—if you want to stock up for later, get a second container, and fill it separately.
3. Fill the container with half-dark greens—lightweight and colorful. Not romaine, which is heavier and therefore can lead to a pricier salad. But tangier greens, such as mesclun, arugula, spinach. Then add at least three different types of colorful raw vegetables. Optional: sprouts (low in calories, but also low in flavor, and often touched with chlorine).
4. Look for lean protein: chunks of tuna, hard-boiled eggs, even diced chicken, cubes of tofu. Add several tablespoons, to cover the lettuce.
5. Avoid anything that is "white" and has the word *salad* attached to the name. This includes anything made with cream cheese, mayonnaise, or sour cream, as well as any premade salads like tuna, chicken, pasta, or potato. These are not high-quality foods, and usually come from a one- or five-gallon container in back.
6. Avoid fruit, unless it is unpeeled and whole; it's hard to know what it has been treated with or soaked in.
7. Skip the premade dressing: use the liquid from the baby corn or the marinated shrimp, or the sliced olives, or an actual avocado or guacamole, thinned with lemon or lime juice or vinegar. Use an oil-and-vinegar dressing, or pure lemon juice, if they have it, and put it in a small dressing container, so you can control the amount, and so your salad does not get soggy. Be liberal with seasonings: I like Braggs Liquid Aminos: meaty, not truly salty, flavorful. Rice, red wine, and balsamic vinegars are tasty, too.
8. Top with seeds for crunch. Not bacon bits (preserved with nitrates), croutons (a rip-off), fried noodles (geez, really?), or tortilla strips (also industrial).

You don't have to be on a cross-country trip to follow these guidelines for eating on the go—even a trip across town can be loaded with food traps and gut bombs. Revisit these tips and stash them in the back pocket of your brain, ready to be recalled when needed. Or, keep this book in your glove compartment, on your dash, or in your briefcase, and mark this page.

WHEN FAST FOOD IS THE ONLY OPTION

A 2011 *Consumer Reports* survey found that less than 20 percent of people felt they got their money's worth from a fast-food establishment. Still, customers pile in—McDonald's alone serves 671 customers per second worldwide.

You're better off not being one of those customers—fast food is filled with aging trans fats, hypertension-inducing levels of sodium, and highly processed carbs and sugars that will drive your insulin up first and boost belly fat shortly thereafter. Fast food and health are like the Yankees and Red Sox—eternal rivals. But you probably know this already. To help flush out the high levels of sodium in these foods, drink plenty of citrus water, or water with lemon with meals—that's one healthy choice you can always make no matter where you stop.

If you must pick up fast food, follow these rules:

1. Ask yourself: how hungry am I? Answer honestly. You might be able to make it to a grocery store just down the road.
2. Never super-size. Ever.
3. Subtract sauces, add vegetables: lettuce, tomato, and onion are likely to be your only options. But they're good.
4. Avoid fried or breaded items, including vegetables. Fried zucchini is not on your list. Ditto onion rings as big as your head.
5. Consider salads, but don't consider them healthy. A grilled chicken salad at Burger King with fat-free dressing has over 1,100 milligrams of sodium.

> **HOT TIP**
> They say good things come in threes. Not burger patties. The Burger King Triple Whopper with cheese has 1,200 calories, 80 grams of fat, and 1,590 milligrams of sodium.

Here are a few items you can eat in a moment of drive-thru desperation.

FAST FOOD FINDS—FOR EMERGENCY USE ONLY					
BURGERS	Calories	Fat	Carbs	Protein	Sodium
Burger King Original Whopper Jr. (no mayo)	310	13g	31g	17g	510mg
McDonald's hamburger	260	9g	33g	13g	530mg
Wendy's Jr. hamburger	280	9g	34g	15g	600mg
MISCELLANEOUS					
Arby's Martha's Vineyard Grilled Chicken Salad	250	8g	23g	26g	490mg
Taco Bell Grilled Steak Soft Tacos (2)	340	10g	42g	22g	560mg
McDonald's Fruit 'N Yogurt Parfait with Granola	160	2g	31g	4g	85mg

> **HOT TIP**
>
> Don't let health claims get into your head. People eating at Subway underestimated their calorie consumption by 27 percent, simply because they thought it was a healthy choice. Before you order, ask for a nutritional fact sheet to see what you're really eating, before you eat it.

ON-THE-JOB EATING

Of course, you don't have to be on a road trip to face the perils of restaurant eating—just heading out the door to work can lead to challenges. Especially because breaks from work usually mean it's time to eat or drink food. We'd be better off if we took road trip breaks to walk or stretch—these activities would relieve stress, ease muscle tightness and tired eyes, and go easier on the wallet.

When Accounting Principals, a Florida-based finance firm, surveyed American workers on their daily spending habits, they discovered some hefty numbers. The average worker spends over $1,092 on coffee alone, and another $1,924 on lunches out. That's enough for a nice vacation and more than you'd need for a down payment on a new car. Economically, it makes sense to pack a lunch from home (yes, you will still spend money at the grocery store, but you get more bang for your buck). Calorie-wise, it's just smart, since eating lunch out has been shown to add 158 extra calories to a person's daily total versus taking lunch from home. The question is: Will you plan to do it? And then do it? Food away from home is almost always more calorically dense than food from home. End of story.

Don't let perfect be the enemy of good. Bring your lunch as often as you can, avoid the break room during seven-layer salad orgies (see "You've Got to Try This," below), and keep your food in your desk drawer. It's smart, too, to take the candy and snacks off your desk: you then avoid being on the see-food diet.

▶ "YOU'VE GOT TO TRY THIS"

My patients often ask how to stick to what they want to eat whenever they come up against pushers—those people who absolutely insist you try their homemade duck confit or triple-fudge macadamia nut cake. Or, what to do when the boss wants to split a pizza? Others want to know how to respond when the mother-in-law packs up all the mac and cheese and brownies "for the kids."

Ultimately, what you eat is up to you. You're in charge, and being confident in your choices is the quickest way to establish your ground.

- **To the pusher in the break room,** say "I'd love to, but I can't." Don't elaborate. Repeat if necessary. Try it—it works.
- **To your boss,** say "I'm going to try this carpaccio and get a bowl of minestrone soup, but the pizza looks good." Still stuck? Say that having food higher in protein makes you a better employee: "I'm more productive and have a lot more energy." Smile when you see him or her yawning during your 2:00 meeting.
- **And to your mother-in-law,** perhaps the most challenging scenario given the goal to always keep the peace, say "Thanks. You're always so generous, but we've got plenty of food prepped for the week." (Even if you don't, and then go home and prep it.) If you absolutely have to take it, even though I hate waste, throw it out as soon as you leave.

Make it easy by anchoring your promises to yourself—for example, each week, try to bring lunch one more time than you did the week prior. Do whatever you need to do to make it happen:

- Bribe your spouse into packing lunch for you.
- Place lunch items in your drawer at work for a whole week, and replenish the next week.
- Put a bagged lunch in front of the doorway at home at night before you go to bed so you run into it and can't forget it.
- Post a temporary "PACK LUNCH" note by your toothbrush; keep it there until it becomes a habit to pack the lunch.

Of course, if possible, go home for lunch. If you want to add a little extra incentive, start a "what's not for lunch" club, and challenge your co-workers to a weight-loss competition.

▸ BEST OFFICE FOODS
(Some snacks are highlighted here for specific use)

BEST BREAKFAST TO EAT IN FRONT OF YOUR MONITOR: Almonds and cheese sticks.

BEST BOTTLED BEVERAGE: Honest Tea's Just Green Tea; it's one-fourth the caffeine of coffee, organic tea, purified water, bottled in glass. No calories.

BEST INSTANT SOUP: Right Foods' Light Sodium Lentil Couscous; it's vegan, gluten-free, high in fiber, high in protein (12 grams), and has no chemical additives. Just 190 calories.

BEST PACKAGED SNACKS: Almonds; Emerald has 100-calorie packs. Sargento String Cheese has just 50 calories and 6 grams of protein.

BEST QUICK-ENERGY SNACK: Organic pumpkin seeds (per ¼ cup) are 180 calories, 9 grams of protein, 4 grams of carbs, and 3 grams of fiber.

BEST SWEET SNACK: Scharffen Berger's Roasted Cacao Nibs; roasted cocoa beans, husked and crushed, with 70 calories per tablespoon, or 130 for 1 ounce; no sugar.

BEST CHOCOLATE BAR: A 99% cacao bar; Cost Plus carries its own line. Lindt Excellence 99% is awesome—takes getting used to, little sugar, and very dark.

BEST READY-TO-EAT PROTEIN BOOST: Bumble Bee Premium Wild Pink Salmon Pouch; a 2-ounce serving has 60 calories, 14 grams of protein, and 2 grams of fat.

BEST MEAL FOR BURNING THE MIDNIGHT OIL: Organic roasted turkey breast with Kashi TLC Snack Crackers Original 7-Grain.

BEST YOGURTS: Chobani, Athenos, and FAGE are all good, high-protein, low- or no-sugar choices among Greek-style (strained, thicker) yogurts; buy unflavored and flavor it yourself.

To prepare to pack lunches at home, pick up a small lunch-size or collapsible cooler and an ice pack that will fit in it. Also, you'll need portable containers—Rubbermaid has some BPA-free options.

When cooking or assembling meals in your kitchen, double or triple the recipe. If your kitchen is the supermarket salad bar, buy double the amount you need. Transfer leftovers directly into travel containers that you can easily grab out of the fridge in the morning.

Eating out is a minefield, and your charge is to avoid detonating the bombs. Refuel is designed to put you in control of your food environment. Find something that works at your favorite restaurant and get it again. Diversity is great, but not when eating out. Once you've learned to take control, you can tinker with your own easy wins to determine how to adjust to the next new place, when you encounter one. Remember that this is an ongoing process, not like flipping a switch. But either way, you can turn the light on.

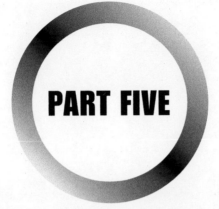

PART FIVE

FINAL THOUGHTS

Men Don't Diet. Men Refuel™.

REFUEL FOR LIFE

The missing link in men's health is the one that physiologically defines men as men: natural testosterone synthesis and use. Too many men are couch-ridden because their bellies have betrayed them: their testes-made testosterone has been switched out for fat-made estrogen. This is not men's fault. The hellish trinity of environmental toxins, crushing economic conditions, and highly processed substances masquerading as food has bulldozed men's health to the side of the road and left it in a ditch to die.

Until now. Because the kitchen can become as crucial as the clinic, being able to provide both health and a healthy weight for yourself and your family is now within the grasp of every man. The simple calories-in, calories-out notion gives us the illusion of being in numerical control of our weight and health. But calories are not all alike; the kind of calories you eat matters.

Refuel aims to be more than a diet program; it aims to be a reward. You can eat for pleasure and become lean. You can restore vitality to your sex drive and recharge your game. The Refuel tools are now in your possession: seize and conquer—in the kitchen, in the bedroom, at the office.

In fact, you're stronger than you think. You don't have to be stuck taking medicines for pain, depression, diabetes, high cholesterol, or high blood pressure forever. You don't have to carry the same risk of heart disease or cancer that your dad or brother or uncle has—or had. You can control your destiny by choosing what you eat. Some men already do.

With just a little guidance—a fraction of what you have here in this book—men who follow Refuel™ begin to see less waist and more of themselves. They experience, in just 24 days, a profound shift in how they want to live and what they want to feel and look like every day. They get a wake-up call, and with it, a realization of what is possible. Even a glimpse of that possibility is enough to make them want more.

Refuel gives you the immediate benefits of eating higher-quality food. Those benefits are personal and powerful—sexual, physical, and muscular. In other words, they are masculine.

I hope that you will use this plan to mark not an end but a beginning. Take 24 days, and turn it into a sea change for your health, for yourself, for your family and loved ones, and for other men and boys around you. Your strength, energy, alertness, and virility will return. You will become more of who you want to be and truly are.

I believe in the power of people to change and reinvent their lives. Refuel instills that power in you. Take it, wield it, share it. It's yours.

REFUEL CARB CHART

Calories count even more than carbs, but to stay within your 50-gram carb days, you have to know what's in what you eat. And your 50-gram carb days are the key to Refuel eating.

REFUEL CARB CHART		
Food	**Serving**	**Carbs**
FISH AND SHELLFISH		
Salmon (Chinook, Coho, or canned)	3 oz (small palm of your hand)	0
Tuna (fresh or canned)	3 oz	0
Flounder	3 oz	0
Halibut	3 oz	0
Shrimp, mixed species, steamed	3 oz	0
MEAT AND POULTRY		
Chicken breast	3 oz	0
Turkey (white or dark meat)	3 oz	0
Beef (ground, extra lean)	3 oz	0

REFUEL CARB CHART (continued)

Food	Serving	Carbs
PORK		
Ham, cured, boneless roasted	3 oz	0
Ham, fresh (leg), lean only, roasted	3 oz	0
SOY PRODUCTS		
Tofu, silken, lite	½ cup	1.5 g
Tofu, firm	½ cup	5.4 g
Edamame, in pods	1 cup	13.5 g
EGG PRODUCTS		
Egg	1 large	0.4 g
Egg white	1 large	0.2 g
Egg yolk	1 large	0.6 g
DAIRY PRODUCTS		
Yogurt, low-fat, plain	1 cup	17.2 g
Yogurt, Greek, plain	1 cup	11.4 g
Cheddar cheese, shredded	½ cup	0.7 g
Mozzarella cheese, part-skim, shredded	½ cup	4.3 g
Feta cheese, crumbled	½ cup	3.0 g
Parmesan cheese, grated	½ cup	2.0 g
Cream cheese	2 tbsp	1.1 g
VEGETABLES		
Celery, chopped, raw	½ cup	1.5 g
Cucumber, peeled	1 small	3.4 g
Mushrooms, slices, raw	½ cup	1.1 g
Romaine lettuce, shredded, raw	1 cup	1.5 g
Asparagus, raw	4 med. spears	2.5 g
Carrot, raw	1 small	4.8 g
Garlic	1 clove	1.0 g
Broccoli, chopped, boiled	½ cup	3.0 g
Cauliflower, chopped, raw	½ cup	2.6 g
Eggplant, cubed, raw	1 cup	4.8 g
Kale, chopped, raw	1 cup	5.9 g
Onion, chopped, raw	½ cup	7.5 g
Spinach, raw	1 cup	1.1 g
Tomato, raw	1 small	3.5 g

REFUEL CARB CHART (continued)

Food	Serving	Carbs
OILS		
Olive oil	I tbsp	0
Canola oil	I tbsp	0
Sesame oil	I tbsp	0
Sunflower oil	I tbsp	0
NUTS AND SEEDS		
Almonds, dry-roasted	I oz (22)	6.0 g
Cashews, dry-roasted	I oz (18)	9.3 g
Pecans, dry-roasted	I oz (19 halves)	3.8 g
Pistachios, dry-roasted	I oz (49)	8.3 g
Walnuts, English	I oz (14 halves)	3.9 g
Sunflower seed kernels	I oz (¼ cup)	5.3 g
Pumpkin seeds, roasted	I oz (85)	4.1 g
FRUITS		
Blueberries, raw	I cup	21.4 g
Strawberries, raw	I cup (whole)	II.I g
Apples, raw	I small (5 oz), with skin	20.5 g
Avocado, all varieties	½ small (3 oz)	7.3 g
Banana	I small (4 oz)	23.I g
Orange	I small (4.5 oz)	14.4 g
Grapes	I cup	15.8 g
Peach	I small (2.5 oz)	12.4 g
Lemon juice	I tbsp	1.3 g
GRAINS, HOT CEREALS, AND PASTA		
Couscous, cooked	½ cup	18.2 g
Rice, brown, cooked	½ cup	22.9 g
Oats, old-fashioned, dry	½ cup	27.0 g
Spaghetti, enriched, cooked	I cup	43.2 g
Spaghetti, whole wheat, cooked	I cup	37.2 g
BREADS		
Bagel	I small	36.8 g
Whole wheat bread	I slice	II.6 g
Pita	I small (4″ diameter)	15.4 g

REFUEL GLOSSARY

ANDROGENS male hormones; androstendione and testosterone are two male hormones.

AROMATASE the enzyme made by fat cells, which converts androgens to estrogens; it turns testosterone to estradiol, the most potent form of estrogen.

ATRAZINE one of the most common commercial herbicides in the United States, with links to obesity and feminization of male reproductive organs.

BISPHENOL-A (BPA) a chemical compound found in polycarbonate plastics and epoxy resins; it's used in all sorts of plastic goods, including water bottles, food packaging, sunglasses, and medical devices.

BURST TRAINING quick bursts of exercise, going nearly all-out followed by longer intervals at a more moderate or mild pace; also known as *interval training, sprint training,* or *high-intensity interval training* (HIIT).

CORTISOL the chronic stress hormone; men make more of it than women, and at a faster rate.

CYTOKINES a class of immunoregulatory proteins similar to hormones made by the immune system.

ENDOCRINE SYSTEM the body's system of internal glands that produce hormones and help to control metabolism.

ESTROGEN a class of feminizing female hormones normally made in tiny amounts by the testes and adrenal glands; estradiol and estrones are both estrogens.

INSULIN the main hormone regulating the blood sugar; made by the islet cells in the pancreas.

INSULIN RESISTANCE the body's subnormal response to normal insulin blood levels and its inability to lower blood sugar; insulin resistance can be caused by too much visceral fat.

LEPTIN a hormone that turns off feelings of hunger; it is made primarily by subcutaneous fat, and women make more leptin than men.

LEPTIN RESISTANCE the result when the body no longer responds to leptin's signal to turn off hunger sensations, causing overeating and confusing the body's system for storing and using energy.

METABOLISM refers to the chemical reactions in the body that lead to creating, using, or storing energy, including making and processing new molecules and cells.

MITOCHONDRIA power plants in your cells inherited only from your mother. Mitochondria make 36 units of energy for every 2 units you get from a sugar molecule.

PERSISTENT ORGANIC POLLUTANT (POP) a blanket term to describe environmental synthetic chemicals and pesticides, including dioxins, polychlorinated biphenyls (PCBs), and organotins; many of these chemicals have been connected to reproductive abnormalities in men.

PHTHALATES (*THAL*-ATES) anti-androgens added to plastics to make them more flexible; used in children's toys, garden hoses, food packaging, toothbrushes, tools, shower curtains, and vinyl flooring; also used in many scented liquid products to help extend the life of the fragrance.

SEX HORMONE–BINDING GLOBULIN (SHBG) a protein made primarily by the liver that binds to testosterone and estradiol in the bloodstream, making them temporarily inactive.

SUBCUTANEOUS FAT the fat you can pinch that's in the love handles; not intensively hormone-producing, like visceral fat.

SYNEPHRINE an organic compound found in the rind and juice of citrus fruits, especially tangerines and sour oranges, which accelerates metabolism; component of Refuel's Citrus Water (page 207).

TESTOSTERONE the main male hormone, produced primarily by the testes, responsible for sex drive, muscle metabolism, strength building, beard presence, and masculinizing characteristics; too much or too little testosterone results in insulin resistance.

VISCERAL FAT surrounds your liver and pancreas, increases your waist size, and sends fatty acids and cytokines straight to the liver to develop insulin resistance.

BIBLIOGRAPHY

CHAPTER 1: THE BIOLOGY OF WEIGHT AND SEX

Bleich, S. N., W. L. Bennett, K. A. Gudzune, and L. A. Cooper. "Impact of Physician BMI on Obesity Care and Beliefs." *Obesity* 20, no. 5 (2012): 999–1005.

Couillard, C., N. Bergeron, et al. "Gender Difference in Postprandial Lipemia." *Arteriosclerosis, Thrombosis, and Vascular Biology* 19, no. 10 (1999): 2448–2455.

Debette, S., A. Beiser, et al. "Visceral Fat Is Associated with Lower Brain Volume in Healthy Middle-Aged Adults." *Annals of Neurology* 68, no. 2 (2010): 136–144.

Dwyer, A. A., L. M. Caronia, et al. "Lifestyle Modification Can Reverse Hypogonadism in Men with Impaired Glucose Tolerance in the Diabetes Prevention Program." ENDO 2012, Endocrine Society 94th Annual Meeting, June 25, 2012. Abstract OR28–3.

Ellem, S. J., and G. P. Risbridger. "Aromatase and Regulating the Estrogen:Androgen Ratio in the Prostate Gland." *Journal of Steroid Biochemistry and Molecular Biology* 118, no. 4–5 (2010): 246–251.

Geer, E. B., and W. Shen. "Gender Differences in Insulin Resistance, Body Composition, and Energy Balance." *Gender Medicine: Official Journal of the Partnership for Gender-Specific Medicine at Columbia University* 6 (2009): 60–75.

Gustafson, B. "Adipose Tissue, Inflammation and Atherosclerosis." *Journal of Atherosclerosis and Thrombosis* 17, no. 4 (2010): 332–341.

Hamdy, O., S. Porramatikul, and E. Al-Ozairi. "Metabolic Obesity: The Paradox Between Visceral and Subcutaneous Fat." *Current Diabetes Reviews* 2, no. 4 (2006): 367–373.

Hayashi, T., E. J. Boyko, et al. "Visceral Adiposity, Not Abdominal Subcutaneous Fat Area, Is Associated with an Increase in Future Insulin Resistance in Japanese Americans." *Diabetes* 57, no. 5 (2008): 1269–1275.

Kaiser Family Foundation, statehealthfacts.org. "Overweight and Obesity Rates for Adults by Gender, 2010." Data Source: Centers for Disease Control and Prevention, Behavioral Risk Factor Surveillance System Survey Data (BRFSS), 2010, unpublished data.

Krotkiewski M., P, Björntorp, L, Sjöström, and U. Smith. "Impact of Obesity on Metabolism in Men and Women." *Journal of Clinical Investigation* 72, no. 3 (1983): 1150–1162. doi:10.1172/JCI111040.

Kuk, J. L., P. T. Katzmarzyk, et al. "Visceral Fat Is an Independent Predictor of All-Cause Mortality in Men." *Obesity* 14, no. 2 (2006): 336–341.

Kvist, H., B. Chowdhury, et al. "Total and Visceral Adipose-Tissue Volumes Derived from Measurements with Computed Tomography in Adult Men and Women: Predictive Equations." *American Journal of Clinical Nutrition* 48, no. 6 (1988): 1351–1361.

LeBlanc, E. S., P. Y. Wang, et al. "Higher Testosterone Levels Are Associated with Less Loss of Lean Body Mass in Older Men." *Journal of Clinical Endocrinology & Metabolism* 96, no. 12 (2011): 3855–3863.

Lemieux, S., D. Prud'homme, et al. "Sex Differences in the Relation of Visceral Adipose Tissue Accumulation to Total Body Fatness." *American Journal of Clinical Nutrition* 58, no. 4 (1993): 463–467.

McTernan, P. G., A. Anwar, et al. "Gender Differences in the Regulation of P450 Aromatase Expression and Activity in Human Adipose Tissue." *International Journal of Obesity* 24, no. 7 (2000): 875–881.

Meindl, K., S. Windhager, et al. "Second-to-Fourth Digit Ratio and Facial Shape in Boys: The Lower the Digit Ratio, the More Robust the Face." *Proceedings of the Royal Society B: Biological Sciences,* February 5, 2012.

Morgan, P., C. Collins, et al. "The SHED-IT Community Trial Study Protocol: A Randomised Controlled Trial of Weight Loss Programs for Overweight and Obese Men." *BMC Public Health* 10, no. 1 (2010): 701.

Morgan, P. J., D. R. Lubans, et al. "The SHED-IT Randomized Controlled Trial: Evaluation of an Internet-Based Weight-Loss Program for Men." *Obesity* 17, no. 11 (2009): 2025–2032.

Murphy S. L., J. Q. Xu, et al. "Deaths: Preliminary Data for 2010." *National Vital Statistics Reports* 60, no 4 (2012).

Ohkawara, K., S. Tanaka, et al. "A Dose-Response Relation Between Aerobic Exercise and Visceral Fat Reduction: Systematic Review of Clinical Trials." *International Journal of Obesity* 31, no. 12 (2008): 1786–1797.

Pischon, T., H. Boeing, K. Hoffmann, et al. "General and Abdominal Adiposity and Risk of Death in Europe." *New England Journal of Medicine* 359, no. 20 (2008): 2105–2120.

Pitteloud, N., V. K. Mootha, et al. "Relationship Between Testosterone Levels, Insulin Sensitivity, and Mitochondrial Function in Men." *Diabetes Care* 28, no. 7 (2005): 1636–1642.

Poulter, J., G. Raine, and S. Robertson. "Evaluation of a Gender-Segregated, Commercial, Community Based, Weight Management Pilot." Supplement, *Obesity Facts* 5, no. S1 (2012): S67.

Ronti, T., G. Lupattelli, et al. "The Endocrine Function of Adipose Tissue: An Update." *Clinical Endocrinology* 64, no. 4 (2006): 355–365.

Van Pelt, R. E., C. M. Jankowski, et al. "Sex Differences in the Association of Thigh Fat and Metabolic Risk in Older Adults." *Obesity* 19, no. 2 (2011): 422–428.

Wang, C., G. Jackson, et al. "Low Testosterone Associated with Obesity and the Metabolic Syndrome Contributes to Sexual Dysfunction and Cardiovascular Disease Risk in Men with Type 2 Diabetes." *Diabetes Care* 34, no. 7 (2011): 1669–1675.

Williams, G. "Aromatase Up-Regulation, Insulin and Raised Intracellular Oestrogens in Men, Induce Adiposity, Metabolic Syndrome and Prostate Disease, Via Aberrant ER-A and GPER Signaling." *Molecular and Cellular Endocrinology* 351, no. 2 (2012): 269–278.

Wu, B. N., and A. J. O'Sullivan. "Sex Differences in Energy Metabolism Need to Be Considered with Lifestyle Modifications in Humans." *Journal of Nutrition and Metabolism,* Article ID 391809 (2011).

CHAPTER 2: TOXINS

Abell, A., E. Ernst, et al. "Semen Quality and Sexual Hormones in Greenhouse Workers." *Scandinavian Journal of Work, Environment and Health* 26, no. 6 (2000): 492–500.

Centers for Disease Control and Prevention. *Fourth Report on Human Exposure to Environmental Chemicals* (2009). http://www.cdc.gov/exposurereport/.

Centers for Disease Control and Prevention. *Fourth Report on Human Exposure to Environmental Chemicals, Updated Tables* (2012). http://www.cdc.gov/exposurereport/.

Desdoits-Lethimonier, C., O. Albert, et al. "Human Testis Steroidogenesis Is Inhibited by Phthalates." *Human Reproduction* (2012). doi:10.1093/humrep/des069.

Diamanti-Kandarakis, E., J.-P. Bourguignon, et al. "Endocrine-Disrupting Chemicals: An Endocrine Society Scientific Statement." *Endocrine Reviews* 30, no. 4 (2009): 293–342.

"Drugs Associated with Weight Gain." *Pharmacist's Letter/Prescriber's Letter* 23, no. 3 (2007): 220312.

Duty, S. M., P. S. Narendra, et al. "The Relationship Between Environmental

Exposures to Phthalates and DNA Damage in Human Sperm Using the Neutral Comet Assay." *Environmental Health Perspectives* 111, no. 9 (2003): 1164–1169.

Hauser, R., and R. Sokol. "Science Linking Environmental Contaminant Exposures with Fertility and Reproductive Health Impacts in the Adult Male." *Fertility and Sterility* 89, no. 2 (2008): e59–e65.

Hauser, R., J. D. Meeker, et al. "Altered Semen Quality in Relation to Urinary Concentrations of Phthalate Monoester and Oxidative Metabolites." *Epidemiology* 17, no. 6 (2006): 682–691.

Hayes, T. B., L. L. Anderson, et al. "Demasculinization and Feminization of Male Gonads by Atrazine: Consistent Effects Across Vertebrate Classes." *Journal of Steroid Biochemistry and Molecular Biology* 127, no. 1–2 (2011): 64–73.

Holtcamp, W. "Obesogens: An Environmental Link to Obesity." *Environmental Health Perspectives* 120 (2012): a62–a68.

Houlihan, J., S. Lunder, et al. "Timeline: BPA from Invention to Phase-Out." Environmental Working Group, last modified March 2011. http://www.ewg.org/reports/bpatimeline.

Kelley, K. E., S. Hernández-Díaz, et al. "Identification of Phthalates in Medications and Dietary Supplement Formulations in the United States and Canada." *Environmental Health Perspectives* 120, no. 3 (2012): 379–384. doi: 10.1289/ehp.1103998.

Kumar, S. "Occupational Exposure Associated with Reproductive Dysfunction." *Journal of Occupational Health* 46, no. 1 (2004): 1–19.

Lee, D.-H., I.-K. Lee, et al. "A Strong Dose-Response Relation Between Serum Concentrations of Persistent Organic Pollutants and Diabetes." *Diabetes Care* 29, no. 7 (2006): 1638–1644.

Li, D.-K., Z. Zhou, et al. "Relationship Between Urine Bisphenol-A Level and Declining Male Sexual Function." *Journal of Andrology* 31, no. 5 (2010): 500–506.

Lim, J. S., H. K. Son, et al. "Inverse Associations Between Long-Term Weight Change and Serum Concentrations of Persistent Organic Pollutants." *International Journal of Obesity* 35, no. 5 (2011): 744–747.

Lim, S., S. Y. Ahn, et al. "Chronic Exposure to the Herbicide, Atrazine, Causes Mitochondrial Dysfunction and Insulin Resistance." *PLoS ONE* 4, no. 4 (2009): e5186.

Lind, P. M., B. van Bavel, et al. "Circulating Levels of Persistent Organic Pollutants (Pops) and Carotid Atherosclerosis in the Elderly." *Environmental Health Perspectives* 120, no. 1 (2012): 38–43.

Porta, M., and L. Duk-Hee. *Review of the Science Linking Chemical Exposures to the Human Risk of Obesity and Diabetes,* CHEMTrust, January 2012.

Reuben, S. H. *Reducing Environmental Cancer Risk: What We Can Do Now. President's Cancer Panel 2008–2009 Annual Report.* Bethesda: National Cancer Institute, 2010.

Rostkowski, P., J. Horwood, et al. "Bioassay-Directed Identification of Novel

Antiandrogenic Compounds in Bile of Fish Exposed to Wastewater Effluents." *Environmental Science & Technology* 45, no. 24 (2011): 10660–10667.

Rudel, R. A., J. M. Gray, et al. "Food Packaging and Bisphenol A and Bis(2-Ethyhexyl) Phthalate Exposure: Findings from a Dietary Intervention." *Environmental Health Perspectives* 119, no. 7 (2011): 914–920.

Ruzzin, J., D.-H. Lee, et al. "Reconsidering Metabolic Diseases: The Impacts of Persistent Organic Pollutants." *Atherosclerosis* 224, no. 1 (2012): 1–3.

Shankar, A., and S. Teppala. "Urinary Bisphenol A and Hypertension in a Multi-ethnic Sample of U.S. Adults." *Journal of Environmental and Public Health,* Article ID 481641 (2012). doi:10.1155/2012/481641.

Slater, D. "The Frog of War." *Mother Jones,* January/February 2012.

Stahlhut R. W., E. van Wijngaarden, et al. "Concentrations of Urinary Phthalate Metabolites Are Associated with Increased Waist Circumference and Insulin Resistance in Adult U.S. Males." *Environmental Health Perspectives* 115, no. 6 (2007): 876–882.

Swan S. H., K. M. Main, et al. "Decrease in Anogenital Distance among Male Infants with Prenatal Phthalate Exposure." *Environmental Health Perspectives* 113 (2005): 1056–1061. http://dx.doi.org/10.1289/ehp.8100.

Wu, M., M. Quirindongo, et al. *Still Poisoning the Well: Atrazine Continues to Contaminate Surface Water and Drinking Water in the United States,* Natural Resources Defense Council, April 2010.

Zoeller, R. T., T. R. Brown, et al. "Endocrine-Disrupting Chemicals and Public Health Protection: A Statement of Principles from the Endocrine Society." *Endocrinology* (2012): 4097–4110.

CHAPTER 3: THE .350 AVERAGE

American Heart Association. "Lack of Sleep May Increase Calorie Consumption." *ScienceDaily,* March 14, 2012. http://www.sciencedaily.com/releases/2012/03/120314170456.htm.

American Psychological Association. *2011 Stress in America Report,* released January 11, 2012. http://www.apa.org/news/press/releases/stress/2011/final-2011.pdf.

Andersen, M. L., and S. Tufik. "The Effects of Testosterone on Sleep and Sleep-Disordered Breathing in Men: Its Bidirectional Interaction with Erectile Function." *Sleep Medicine Reviews* 12, no. 5 (2008): 365–379.

Ayas, N. T. "If You Weigh Too Much, Maybe You Should Try Sleeping More." *Sleep* 33, no. 2 (2010): 143–144.

Barrett-Connor, E., T.-T. Dam, et al. "The Association of Testosterone Levels with Overall Sleep Quality, Sleep Architecture, and Sleep-Disordered Breathing." *Journal of Clinical Endocrinology & Metabolism* 93, no. 7 (2008): 2602–2609.

Bartlett, J. D., G. L. Close, et al. "High-Intensity Interval Running Is Perceived to Be More Enjoyable Than Moderate-Intensity Continuous Exercise: Implications for Exercise Adherence." *Journal of Sports Sciences* 29, no. 6 (2011): 547–553.

Benedict, C., S. J. Brooks, et al. "Acute Sleep Deprivation Enhances the Brain's Response to Hedonic Food Stimuli: An fMRI Study." *Journal of Clinical Endocrinology & Metabolism* (2012): E1–E5.

Brody, S. "Blood Pressure Reactivity to Stress Is Better for People Who Recently Had Penile–Vaginal Intercourse Than for People Who Had Other or No Sexual Activity." *Biological Psychology* 71, no. 2 (2006): 214–222.

Burgess, H. J., J. Trinder, et al. "Sleep and Circadian Influences on Cardiac Autonomic Nervous System Activity." *American Journal of Physiology–Heart and Circulatory Physiology* 273, no. 4 (1997): H1761–H1768.

Cappuccio, F. P., F. M. Taggart, et al. "Meta-Analysis of Short Sleep Duration and Obesity in Children and Adults." *Sleep* 31, no. 5 (2008): 619–626.

Chellappa, S. L., A. U. Viola, et al. "Human Melatonin and Alerting Response to Blue-Enriched Light Depend on a Polymorphism in the Clock Gene PER3." *Journal of Clinical Endocrinology & Metabolism* 97, no. 3 (2012): E433–E437.

Conroy, D. E., S. Elavsky, et al. "The Dynamic Nature of Physical Activity Intentions: A Within-Person Perspective on Intention-Behavior Coupling." *Journal of Sport & Exercise Psychology* 33 (2011): 807–827.

Damodaran A., A. Malathi, et al. "Therapeutic Potential of Yoga Practices in Modifying Cardiovascular Risk Profile in Middle Aged Men and Women." *Journal of Association of Physicians of India* 50 (2002): 633–640.

Epel, E. E., A. E. Moyer, et al. "Stress-Induced Cortisol, Mood, and Fat Distribution in Men." *Obesity Research* 7, no. 1 (1999): 9–15.

Felsing, N. E., J. A. Brasel, et al. "Effect of Low and High Intensity Exercise on Circulating Growth Hormone in Men." *Journal of Clinical Endocrinology & Metabolism* 75, no. 1 (1992): 157–162.

Granath, J., S. Ingvarsson, et al. "Stress Management: A Randomized Study of Cognitive Behavioural Therapy and Yoga." *Cognitive Behaviour Therapy* 35, no. 1 (2006): 3–10.

He, C., M. C. Bassik, et al. "Exercise-Induced BCL2-Regulated Autophagy Is Required for Muscle Glucose Homeostasis." *Nature* 481, no. 7382 (2012): 511–515.

Healy, G. N., C. E. Matthews, et al. "Sedentary Time and Cardio-Metabolic Biomarkers in U.S. Adults: NHANES 2003–06." *European Heart Journal* 32, no. 5 (2011): 590–597.

Henderson, G. C., J. A. Fattor, et al. "Lipolysis and Fatty Acid Metabolism in Men and Women During the Postexercise Recovery Period." *Journal of Physiology* 584, no. 3 (2007): 963–981.

Heydari, M., J. Freund, et al. "The Effect of High-Intensity Intermittent Exercise on Body Composition of Overweight Young Males." *Journal of Obesity,* Article ID 480467 (2012). doi:10.1155/2012/480467.

Hiestand, D. M., P. Britz, et al. "Prevalence of Symptoms and Risk of Sleep Apnea in the U.S. Population: Results from the National Sleep Foundation Sleep in America 2005 Poll." *CHEST* 130, no. 3 (2006): 780–786.

Khoo, J., R. Chen, et al. "Comparing Effects of Weight Loss on Sexual, Urinary and Endothelial Function, Insulin Resistance and Quality of Life in Obese Men with and Without Erectile Dysfunction." *Endocrine Abstracts* 29 (2012): P1023.

Kripke, D. F., R. D. Langer, et al. "Hypnotics' Association with Mortality or Cancer: A Matched Cohort Study." *British Medical Journal Open* 2, no. 1 (2012): e000850. doi:10.1136/bmjopen-2012–000850.

Leproult, R., and E. Van Cauter. "Effect of 1 Week of Sleep Restriction on Testosterone Levels in Young Healthy Men." *JAMA: The Journal of the American Medical Association* 305, no. 21 (2011): 2173.

Mayo, M. J., J. R. Grantham, et al. "Exercise-Induced Weight Loss Preferentially Reduces Abdominal Fat." *Medicine & Science in Sports & Exercise* 35, no. 2 (2003): 207–213.

Minkel, J. D., S. Banks, et al. "Sleep Deprivation and Stressors: Evidence for Elevated Negative Affect in Response to Mild Stressors When Sleep Deprived." *Emotion*, February 6, 2012. doi: 10.1037/a0026871.

Mourier A., J. F. Gautier, et al. "Mobilization of Visceral Adipose Tissue Related to the Improvement in Insulin Sensitivity in Response to Physical Training in NIDDM. Effects of Branched-Chain Amino Acid Supplements." *Diabetes Care* 20, no. 3 (1997): 385–391.

National Sleep Foundation. "Healthy Sleep Tips," accessed September 19, 2012, http://www.sleepfoundation.org/article/sleep-topics/healthy-sleep-tips.

National Sleep Foundation. *Sleep in America Poll, 2011.* Washington, DC: National Sleep Foundation, March 2011.

Onat, A., G. Hergenç, et al. "Neck Circumference as a Measure of Central Obesity: Associations with Metabolic Syndrome and Obstructive Sleep Apnea Syndrome Beyond Waist Circumference." *Clinical Nutrition* 28, no. 1 (2009): 46–51.

Passos, G. S., D. Poyares, et al. "Effects of Moderate Aerobic Exercise Training on Chronic Primary Insomnia." *Sleep Medicine* 12, no. 10 (2011): 1018–1027.

Rosmond, R., and P. Björntorp. "Occupational Status, Cortisol Secretory Pattern, and Visceral Obesity in Middle-Aged Men." *Obesity Research* 8, no. 6 (2000): 445–450.

Schwarz, N. A., B. R. Rigby, et al. "A Review of Weight Control Strategies and Their Effects on the Regulation of Hormonal Balance." *Journal of Nutrition and Metabolism,* Article ID 237932 (2011).

Slentz, C. A., L. B. Aiken, et al. "Inactivity, Exercise, and Visceral Fat. STRRIDE: A Randomized, Controlled Study of Exercise Intensity and Amount." *Journal of Applied Physiology* 99, no. 4 (2005): 1613–1618.

Steptoe, A., S. R. Kunz-Ebrecht, et al. "Central Adiposity and Cortisol Responses to Waking in Middle-Aged Men and Women." *International Journal of Obesity* 28, no. 9 (2004): 1168–1173.

Thompson, D., F. Karpe, et al. "Physical Activity and Exercise in the Regulation of Human Adipose Tissue Physiology." *Physiological Reviews* 92, no. 1 (2012): 157–191.

Van Cauter, E., K. Knutson, et. al. "The Impact of Sleep Deprivation on Hormones and Metabolism." *Medscape Neurology* 7, no. 1 (2005).

Van Cauter, E., K. Spiegel, et al. "Metabolic Consequences of Sleep and Sleep Loss." *Sleep Medicine* 9, supplement 1 (2008): S23–28.

Van Dongen, H. P., G. Maislin, et al. "The Cumulative Cost of Additional Wakefulness: Dose-Response Effects on Neurobehavioral Functions and Sleep Physiology from Chronic Sleep Restriction and Total Sleep Deprivation." *Sleep* 26, no. 2 (2003): 117–126.

Wallerius, S., R. Rosmond, et al. "Rise in Morning Saliva Cortisol Is Associated with Abdominal Obesity in Men: A Preliminary Report." *Journal of Endocrinological Investigation* 26, no. 7 (2003): 616–619.

Watanabe, M., H. Kikuchi, et al. "Association of Short Sleep Duration with Weight Gain and Obesity at 1-Year Follow-Up: A Large-Scale Prospective Study." *Sleep* 33, no. 2 (2010): 161–167.

Wheaton, A., G. Perry, et al. "Relationship Between Body Mass Index and Perceived Insufficient Sleep Among U.S. Adults: An Analysis of 2008 BRFSS Data." *BMC Public Health* 11, no. 1 (2011): 295.

Wolfe, R. R. "The Underappreciated Role of Muscle in Health and Disease." *American Journal of Clinical Nutrition* 84, no. 3 (2006): 475–482.

Zhang J., R. C. Ma, et al. "Relationship of Sleep Quantity and Quality with 24-Hour Urinary Catecholamines and Salivary Awakening Cortisol in Healthy Middle-Aged Adults." *Sleep* 34, no. 2 (2011): 225–233.

CHAPTER 4: THREE QUIZZES

Aeberli, I., P. A. Gerber, et al. "Low To Moderate Sugar-Sweetened Beverage Consumption Impairs Glucose and Lipid Metabolism and Promotes Inflammation in Healthy Young Men: A Randomized Controlled Trial." *American Journal of Clinical Nutrition* 94, no. 2 (2011): 479–485.

Agledahl, I., P.-A. Skjærpe, et al. "Low Serum Testosterone in Men Is Inversely Associated with Non-Fasting Serum Triglycerides: The Tromsø Study." *Nutrition, Metabolism and Cardiovascular Diseases* 18, no. 4 (2008): 256–262.

Brondel, L., M. A. Romer, et al. "Acute Partial Sleep Deprivation Increases Food Intake in Healthy Men." *American Journal of Clinical Nutrition* 91, no. 6 (2010): 1550–1559.

Buxton, O. M., M. Pavlova, et al. "Sleep Restriction for 1 Week Reduces Insulin Sensitivity in Healthy Men." *Diabetes* 59, no. 9 (2010): 2126–2133.

Centers for Disease Control and Prevention. "Lung Cancer Statistics," last updated April 30, 2012. http://www.cdc.gov/cancer/lung/statistics/.

Cooper, J. E., E. L. Kendig, et al. "Assessment of Bisphenol A Released from Reusable Plastic, Aluminium and Stainless Steel Water Bottles." *Chemosphere* 85, no. 6 (2011): 943–947.

Duffey, K. J., P. Gordon-Larsen, et al. "Regular Consumption from Fast Food Establishments Relative to Other Restaurants Is Differentially Associated with Metabolic Outcomes in Young Adults." *Journal of Nutrition* 139, no. 11 (2009): 2113–2118.

Elbaz, A., J. Clavel, et al. "Professional Exposure to Pesticides and Parkinson Disease." *Annals of Neurology* 66, no. 4 (2009): 494–504.

Empen, K., R. Lorbeer, et al. "Association of Testosterone Levels with Endothelial Function in Men." *Arteriosclerosis, Thrombosis, and Vascular Biology* 32, no. 2 (2012): 481–486.

Fink, H. A., S. K. Ewing, et al. "Association of Testosterone and Estradiol Deficiency with Osteoporosis and Rapid Bone Loss in Older Men." *Journal of Clinical Endocrinology & Metabolism* 91, no. 10 (2006): 3908–3915.

Fulkerson, J. A., K. Farbakhsh, et al. "Away-from-Home Family Dinner Sources and Associations with Weight Status, Body Composition, and Related Biomarkers of Chronic Disease Among Adolescents and Their Parents." *Journal of the American Dietetic Association* 111, no. 12 (2011): 1892–1897.

Ganji, V., X. Zhang, et al. "Serum 25-Hydroxyvitamin D Concentrations and Prevalence Estimates of Hypovitaminosis D in the U.S. Population Based on Assay-Adjusted Data." *Journal of Nutrition* 142, no. 3 (2012): 498–507.

Garcia, G., T. Sunil, et al. "The Fast Food and Obesity Link: Consumption Patterns and Severity of Obesity." *Obesity Surgery* 22, no. 5 (2012): 810–818.

Hardin, J., I. Cheng, et al. "Impact of Consumption of Vegetable, Fruit, Grain, and High Glycemic Index Foods on Aggressive Prostate Cancer Risk." *Nutrition and Cancer* 63, no. 6 (2011): 860–872.

Haring, R., S. E. Baumeister, et al. "Prospective Association of Low Total Testosterone Concentrations with an Adverse Lipid Profile and Increased Incident Dyslipidemia." *European Journal of Cardiovascular Prevention & Rehabilitation* 18, no. 1 (2011): 86–96.

Harris, E., J. Kirk, et al. "The Effect of Multivitamin Supplementation on Mood and Stress in Healthy Older Men." *Human Psychopharmacology: Clinical and Experimental* 26, no. 8 (2011): 560–567.

Johnson, L. K., D. Hofso, et al. "Impact of Gender on Vitamin D Deficiency in Morbidly Obese Patients: A Cross-Sectional Study." *European Journal of Clinical Nutrition* 66, no. 1 (2012): 83–90.

Mancia, G., M. Bombelli, et al. "Long-Term Risk of Sustained Hypertension in White-Coat or Masked Hypertension." *Hypertension* 54, no. 2 (2009): 226–232.

Meldrum, D. R., J. C. Gambone, et al. "The Link Between Erectile and Cardiovascular Health: The Canary in the Coal Mine." *American Journal of Cardiology* 108, no. 4 (2011): 599–606.

Mozaffarian, D., J. S. Gottdiener, et al. "Intake of Tuna or Other Broiled or Baked Fish Versus Fried Fish and Cardiac Structure, Function, and Hemodynamics." *American Journal of Cardiology* 97, no. 2 (2006): 216–222.

Mozaffarian, D., T. Hao, et al. "Changes in Diet and Lifestyle and Long-Term Weight Gain in Women and Men." *New England Journal of Medicine* 364, no. 25 (2011): 2392–2404.

National Cancer Institute. "Acrylamide in Food and Cancer Risk," last updated July 2008. http://www.cancer.gov/cancertopics/factsheet/Risk/acrylamide-in-food#r2.

O'Toole, T. E., D. J. Conklin, and A. Bhatnagar. "Environmental Risk Factors for Heart Disease." *Reviews on Environmental Health* 23, no. 3 (2008): 167–202.

Palazoğlu, T. K., D. Savran, et al. "Effect of Cooking Method (Baking Compared with Frying) on Acrylamide Level of Potato Chips." *Journal of Food Science* 75, no. 1 (2010): E25–E29.

Paolo, B., and S. Kurt. "Use of Smokeless Tobacco and Risk of Myocardial Infarction and Stroke: Systematic Review with Meta-Analysis." *British Medical Journal* 339 (2009): b3060.

Pereira, M. A., A. I. Kartashov, et al. "Fast-Food Habits, Weight Gain, and Insulin Resistance (the CARDIA Study): 15-Year Prospective Analysis." *The Lancet* 365, no. 9453 (2005): 36–42.

Rosenheck, R. "Fast Food Consumption and Increased Caloric Intake: A Systematic Review of a Trajectory Towards Weight Gain and Obesity Risk." *Obesity Reviews* 9, no. 6 (2008): 535–547.

Sayon-Orea, C., M. Bes-Rastrollo, et al. "Consumption of Fried Foods and Weight Gain in a Mediterranean Cohort: The SUN Project." *Nutrition, Metabolism and Cardiovascular Diseases,* August 2011. http://dx.doi.org/10.1016/j.numecd.2011.03.014.

Shivpuri, S., L. Gallo, et al. "The Association Between Chronic Stress Type and C-Reactive Protein in the Multi-Ethnic Study of Atherosclerosis: Does Gender Make a Difference?" *Journal of Behavioral Medicine* 35, no. 1 (2012): 74–85.

Sifakis, S., M. Mparmpas, et al. "Pesticide Exposure and Health Related Issues in Male and Female Reproductive System." In *Pesticides—Formulations, Effects, Fate,* edited by Margarita Stoytcheva. Rijeka: InTech, 2011. 495–526.

Svartberg, J., D. von Muhlen, et al. "Association of Endogenous Testosterone with Blood Pressure and Left Ventricular Mass in Men. The Tromso Study." *European Journal of Endocrinology* 150, no. 1 (2004): 65–71.

Tuck, S. P., and R. M. Francis. "Testosterone, Bone and Osteoporosis." *Frontiers of Hormone Research* 37 (2009): 123–132.

Van Leeuwen, W. M. A., C. Hublin, et al. "Prolonged Sleep Restriction Affects Glucose Metabolism in Healthy Young Men." *International Journal of Endocrinology,* Article ID 108641 (2010).

CHAPTER 5: A PLATE FOR TWO

Falba, T. A., and J. L. Sindelar. "Spousal Concordance in Health Behavior Change." *Health Services Research* 43, no. 1p1 (2008): 96–116.

Gough, B. "Try to Be Healthy, but Don't Forgo Your Masculinity: Deconstructing Men's Health Discourse in the Media." *Social Science & Medicine* 63, no. 9 (2006): 2476–2488.

Mahalik, J. R., S. M. Burns, et al. "Masculinity and Perceived Normative Health

Behaviors as Predictors of Men's Health Behaviors." *Social Science & Medicine* 64, no. 11 (2007): 2201–2209.

Mróz, L. W., G. E. Chapman, et al. "Men, Food, and Prostate Cancer: Gender Influences on Men's Diets." *American Journal of Men's Health* 5, no. 2 (2011): 177–187.

Rozin, P., J. M. Hormes, et al. "Is Meat Male? A Quantitative Multimethod Framework to Establish Metaphoric Relationships." *Journal of Consumer Research* 39, no. 3 (2012): 629–643.

Steim, R. I., and C. J. Nemeroff. "Moral Overtones of Food: Judgments of Others Based on What They Eat." *Personality and Social Psychology Bulletin* 21, no. 5 (1995): 480–490.

Stibbe, A. "Health and the Social Construction of Masculinity in *Men's Health* Magazine." *Men and Masculinities* 7, no. 1 (2004): 31–51.

The, N. S., and P. Gordon-Larsen. "Entry into Romantic Partnership Is Associated with Obesity." *Obesity* 17, no. 7 (2009): 1441–1447.

Vartanian, L. R., C. P. Herman, et al. "Consumption Stereotypes and Impression Management: How You Are What You Eat." *Appetite* 48, no. 3 (2007): 265–277.

CHAPTER 7: REFUEL NUTS AND BOLTS

Bernstein, A. M., A. Pan, et al. "Dietary Protein Sources and the Risk of Stroke in Men and Women." *Stroke* 43, no. 3 (2012): 637–644.

Bray, G., S. R. Smith, et al. "Effect of Dietary Protein Content on Weight Gain, Energy Expenditure, and Body Composition During Overeating: A Randomized Controlled Trial." *JAMA: The Journal of the American Medical Association* 307, no. 1 (2012): 47–55.

Cohen, P. G. "Obesity in Men: The Hypogonadal–Estrogen Receptor Relationship and Its Effect on Glucose Homeostasis." *Medical Hypotheses* 70, no. 2 (2008): 358–360.

Gurrola-Díaz, C. M., P. M. García-López, et al. "Effects of Hibiscus Sabdariffa Extract Powder and Preventive Treatment (Diet) on the Lipid Profiles of Patients with Metabolic Syndrome (Mesy)." *Phytomedicine* 17, no. 7 (2010): 500–505.

Harvie, M. N., M. Pegington, et al. "The Effects of Intermittent or Continuous Energy Restriction on Weight Loss and Metabolic Disease Risk Markers: A Randomized Trial in Young Overweight Women." *International Journal of Obesity* 35, no. 5 (2011): 714–727.

Hollis, J. F., C. M. Gullion, et al. "Weight Loss During the Intensive Intervention Phase of the Weight-Loss Maintenance Trial." *American Journal of Preventive Medicine* 35, no. 2 (2008): 118–126.

Karnani, Mahesh M., J. Apergis-Schoute, et al. "Activation of Central Orexin/Hypocretin Neurons by Dietary Amino Acids." *Neuron* 72, no. 4 (2011): 616–629.

Pan A., Q. Sun, et al. "Red Meat Consumption and Mortality: Results from 2 Prospective Cohort Studies." *Archives of Internal Medicine* 172, no. 7 (2012): 555–563.

Siri-Tarino, P. W., Q. Sun, et al. "Meta-Analysis of Prospective Cohort Studies Evaluating the Association of Saturated Fat with Cardiovascular Disease." *American Journal of Clinical Nutrition* 91, no. 3 (2010): 535–546.

Symons, T. B., M. Sheffield-Moore, et al. "A Moderate Serving of High-Quality Protein Maximally Stimulates Skeletal Muscle Protein Synthesis in Young and Elderly Subjects." *Journal of the American Dietetic Association* 109, no. 9 (2009): 1582–1586.

Tey, S. L., R. Brown, et al. "Nuts Improve Diet Quality Compared to Other Energy-Dense Snacks While Maintaining Body Weight." *Journal of Nutrition and Metabolism,* Article ID 357350 (2011).

Wansink, B. "Under the Influence: How External Cues Make Us Overeat." An interview by Bonnie Liebman. *Nutrition Action Health Letter* 3, no. 2 (2011): 3–7.

Watanabe, M., H. Kikuchi, et al. "Association of Short Sleep Duration with Weight Gain and Obesity at 1-Year Follow-Up: A Large-Scale Prospective Study." *Sleep* 33, no. 2 (2010): 161–167.

Williams, G. "Aromatase Up-Regulation, Insulin and Raised Intracellular Oestrogens in Men, Induce Adiposity, Metabolic Syndrome and Prostate Disease, via Aberrant ER-A and GPER Signalling." *Molecular and Cellular Endocrinology* 351, no. 2 (2012): 269–278.

CHAPTER 8: PHASE 1

Aggarwal, B. B. "Targeting Inflammation-Induced Obesity and Metabolic Diseases by Curcumin and Other Nutraceuticals." *Annual Review of Nutrition* 30 (2010): 173–199.

Bernstein, A. M., L. de Koning, et al. "Soda Consumption and the Risk of Stroke in Men and Women." *American Journal of Clinical Nutrition* 95, no. 5 (2012): 1190–1199.

Cajochen, C., S. Frey, et al. "Evening Exposure to Light-Emitting Diodes (LED)— Backlit Computer Screen Affects Circadian Physiology and Cognitive Performance." *Journal of Applied Physiology* 110, no. 5 (2011): 1432–1438.

Chang, C., J. Choi, et al. "Correlation Between Serum Testosterone Level and Concentrations of Copper and Zinc in Hair Tissue." *Biological Trace Element Research* 144, no. 1 (2011): 264–271.

Choi, Y., Y. Kim, et al. "Indole-3-Carbinol Prevents Diet-Induced Obesity Through Modulation of Multiple Genes Related to Adipogenesis, Thermogenesis or Inflammation in the Visceral Adipose Tissue of Mice." *Journal of Nutritional Biochemistry,* May 2012. doi:10.1016/j.jnutbio.2011.12.005.

Cudennec, B., M. Fouchereau-Peron, et al. "In Vitro and In Vivo Evidence for a Satiating Effect of Fish Protein Hydrolysate Obtained from Blue Whiting (Micromesistius Poutassou) Muscle." *Journal of Functional Foods* 4, no. 1 (2012): 271–277.

de Koning, L., V. S. Malik, et al. "Sugar-Sweetened and Artificially Sweetened Beverage Consumption and Risk of Type 2 Diabetes in Men." *American Journal of Clinical Nutrition* 93, no. 6 (2011): 1321–1327.

Duffy, J. F., S. W. Cain, et al. "Sex Difference in the Near-24-Hour Intrinsic Period of the Human Circadian Timing System." *Proceedings of the National Academy of Sciences of the United States of America* 108, supplement 3 (2011): 15602–15608.

Goree, L. L., P. Chandler-Laney, et al. "Dietary Macronutrient Composition Affects B Cell Responsiveness but Not Insulin Sensitivity." *American Journal of Clinical Nutrition* 94, no. 1 (2011): 120–127.

Handjieva-Darlenska, T., S. Handjiev, et al. "Initial Weight Loss on an 800-Kcal Diet as a Predictor of Weight Loss Success After 8 Weeks: The Diogenes Study." *European Journal of Clinical Nutrition* 64, no. 9 (2010): 994–999.

Hsu, C.-L., and G.-C. Yen. "Effects of Capsaicin on Induction of Apoptosis and Inhibition of Adipogenesis in 3T3-L1 Cells." *Journal of Agricultural and Food Chemistry* 55, no. 5 (2007): 1730–1736.

Jemal, A., F. Bray, et al. "Global Cancer Statistics." *A Cancer Journal for Clinicians* 61, no. 2 (March/April 2011): 1542–4863.

Kurahashi, N., S. Sasazuki, et al. "Green Tea Consumption and Prostate Cancer Risk in Japanese Men: A Prospective Study." *American Journal of Epidemiology* 167, no. 1 (2008): 71–77.

Laughlin, G. A., E. Barrett-Connor, et al. "Low Serum Testosterone and Mortality in Older Men." *Journal of Clinical Endocrinology & Metabolism* 93, no. 1 (2008): 68–75.

Lejeune, M. P., E. M. Kovacs, and M. S. Westerterp-Plantenga. "Effect of Capsaicin on Substrate Oxidation and Weight Maintenance After Modest Body-Weight Loss in Human Subjects." *British Journal of Nutrition* 90, no. 3 (2003): 651–659.

Maersk M., A. Belza, et al. "Sucrose-Sweetened Beverages Increase Fat Storage in the Liver, Muscle, and Visceral Fat Depot: A 6-Mo Randomized Intervention Study." *American Journal of Clinical Nutrition* 95, no. 2 (2012): 283–289.

Mekary, R. A., E. Giovannucci, et al. "Eating Patterns and Type 2 Diabetes Risk in Men: Breakfast Omission, Eating Frequency, and Snacking." *American Journal of Clinical Nutrition* 95, no. 5 (2012): 1182–1189.

Meyer, M. R., D. J. Clegg, et al. "Obesity, Insulin Resistance and Diabetes: Sex Differences and Role of Oestrogen Receptors." *Acta Physiologica* 203, no. 1 (2011): 259–269.

Nagao T., T. Hase, et al. "A Green Tea Extract High in Catechins Reduces Body Fat and Cardiovascular Risks in Humans." *Obesity,* no. 6 (2007): 1473–1483.

Nagao, T., Y. Komine, et al. "Ingestion of a Tea Rich in Catechins Leads to a Reduction in Body Fat and Malondialdehyde-Modified LDL in Men." *American Journal of Clinical Nutrition* 81, no. 1 (2005): 122–129.

Park, S.-Y., S. P. Murphy, et al. "Calcium, Vitamin D, and Dairy Product Intake and Prostate Cancer Risk." *American Journal of Epidemiology* 166, no. 11 (2007): 1259–1269.

Pollock, N. K., V. Bundy, et al. "Greater Fructose Consumption Is Associated with Cardiometabolic Risk Markers and Visceral Adiposity in Adolescents." *Journal of Nutrition* 142, no. 2 (2012): 251–257.

Prasad, A. S., C. S. Mantzoros, et al. "Zinc Status and Serum Testosterone Levels of Healthy Adults." *Nutrition* 12, no. 5 (1996): 344–348.

Ruige, J. B., M. Bekaert, et al. "Sex Steroid–Induced Changes in Circulating Monocyte Chemoattractant Protein-1 Levels May Contribute to Metabolic Dysfunction in Obese Men." *Journal of Clinical Endocrinology & Metabolism* 97, no. 7 (2012): E1187–1191.

Sartor, F., M. Jackson, et al. "Adaptive Metabolic Response to 4 Weeks of Sugar-Sweetened Beverage Consumption in Healthy, Lightly Active Individuals and Chronic High Glucose Availability in Primary Human Myotubes." *European Journal of Nutrition* 52, no. 3 (2013). doi:10.1007/s00394–012–0401.

Solomon, T., and A. Blannin. "Changes in Glucose Tolerance and Insulin Sensitivity Following 2 Weeks of Daily Cinnamon Ingestion in Healthy Humans." *European Journal of Applied Physiology* 105, no. 6 (2009): 969–976.

Venditti, E., T. Bacchetti, et al. "Hot vs. Cold Water Steeping of Different Teas: Do They Affect Antioxidant Activity?" *Food Chemistry* 119, no. 4 (2010): 1597–604.

CHAPTER 9: PHASE 2

Cook, D. M., K. C. Yuen, et al. "American Association of Clinical Endocrinologists Medical Guidelines for Clinical Practice for Growth Hormone Use in Growth Hormone–Deficient Adults and Transition Patients—2009 Update." *Endocrine Practice* 15, sup. 2 (2009): 1–29.

Denny-Brown, S., T. L. Stanley, et al. "The Association of Macro- and Micronutrient Intake with Growth Hormone Secretion." *Growth Hormone & IGF Research* 22, no. 3–4 (2012): 102–107.

Lanzi, R., L. Luzi, et al. "Elevated Insulin Levels Contribute to the Reduced Growth Hormone (GH) Response to GH-Releasing Hormone in Obese Subjects." *Metabolism* 48, no. 9 (1999): 1152–1156.

Lanzi, R., M. F. Manzoni, et al. "Evidence for an Inhibitory Effect of Physiological Levels of Insulin on the Growth Hormone (GH) Response to GH-Releasing Hormone in Healthy Subjects." *Journal of Clinical Endocrinology & Metabolism* 82, no. 7 (1997): 2239–2243.

Makimura, H., T. Stanley, et al. "The Effects of Central Adiposity on Growth Hormone (GH) Response to GH-Releasing Hormone-Arginine Stimulation Testing in Men." *Journal of Clinical Endocrinology & Metabolism* 93, no. 11 (2008): 4254–4260.

Norat, T., S. Bingham, et al. "Meat, Fish, and Colorectal Cancer Risk: The European Prospective Investigation into Cancer and Nutrition." *Journal of the National Cancer Institute* 97, no. 12 (2005): 906–916.

Vahl, N., J. O. Jorgensen, et al. "Abdominal Adiposity Rather Than Age and Sex Predicts Mass and Regularity of GH Secretion in Healthy Adults." *American Journal of Physiology—Endocrinology and Metabolism* 272, no. 6 (1997): E1108–E1116.

CHAPTER 10: PHASE 3

Baron, K. G., K. J. Reid, et al. "Role of Sleep Timing in Caloric Intake and BMI." *Obesity* 19, no. 7 (2011): 1374–1381.

Connors, S. K., G. Chornokur, et al. "New Insights into the Mechanisms of Green Tea Catechins in the Chemoprevention of Prostate Cancer." *Nutrition and Cancer* 64, no. 1 (2012): 4–22.

Kwon, J. Y., S. G. Seo, et al. "Piceatannol, Natural Polyphenolic Stilbene, Inhibits Adipogenesis via Modulation of Mitotic Clonal Expansion and Insulin Receptor–Dependent Insulin Signaling in Early Phase of Differentiation." *Journal of Biological Chemistry* 287, no. 14 (2012): 11566–11578.

Puetz, T. W., P. J. O'Connor, et al. "Effects of Chronic Exercise on Feelings of Energy and Fatigue: A Quantitative Synthesis." *Psychological Bulletin* 132, no. 6 (2006): 866–876.

Timmers, S., E. Konings, et al. "Calorie Restriction-like Effects of 30 Days of Resveratrol Supplementation on Energy Metabolism and Metabolic Profile in Obese Humans." *Cell Metabolism* 14, no. 5 (2011): 612–622.

Watson, N. F., K. P. Harden, et al. "Sleep Duration and Body Mass Index in Twins: A Gene-Environment Interaction." *Sleep* 35, no. 5 (2012): 597–603.

CHAPTER 11: THE REFUEL SUPPLEMENT GUIDE

Anderson, J. S., J. A. Nettleton, et al. "Associations of Plasma Phospholipid Omega-6 and Omega-3 Polyunsaturated Fatty Acid Levels and MRI Measures of Cardiovascular Structure and Function: The Multiethnic Study of Atherosclerosis." *Journal of Nutrition and Metabolism,* Article ID 315134 (2011).

Aubrey, A. "The Average American Ate (Literally) a Ton This Year." *The Salt* (NPR's Food Blog), December 31, 2011. http://www.npr.org/blogs/thesalt /2011/12/31/144478009/the-average-american-ate-literally-a-ton-this-year.

Johnson, L. K., D. Hofso, et al. "Impact of Gender on Vitamin D Deficiency in Morbidly Obese Patients: A Cross-Sectional Study." *European Journal of Clinical Nutrition* 66, no. 1 (2012): 83–90.

Lee, D. M., A. Tajar, et al. "Association of Hypogonadism with Vitamin D Status: The European Male Ageing Study." *European Journal of Endocrinology* 166, no. 1 (2012): 77–85.

Park, K., E. B. Rimm, et al. "Toenail Selenium and Incidence of Type 2 Diabetes Mellitus in U.S. Men and Women." *Diabetes Care* 35, no. 7 (2012): 1544–1551.

CHAPTER 12: COOKING IS FREEDOM

Smith, J. S., F. Ameri, et al. "Effect of Marinades on the Formation of Heterocyclic Amines in Grilled Beef Steaks." *Journal of Food Science* 73, no. 6 (2008): T100–T105.

CHAPTER 13: SEE, TASTE, EAT

Neff, J. "Time to Rethink Your Message: Now the Cart Belongs to Daddy." *Advertising Age*, January 17, 2011. http://adage.com/article/news/men-main -grocery-shoppers-complain-ads/148252/.

Wang, G. -J., N. D. Volkow, et al. "Evidence of Gender Differences in the Ability to Inhibit Brain Activation Elicited by Food Stimulation." *Proceedings of the National Academy of Sciences* 106, no. 4 (2009): 1249–1254.

Wansink, B. "Environmental Factors That Increase the Food Intake and Consumption Volume of Unknowing Consumers." *Annual Review of Nutrition* 24, no. 1 (2004): 455–479.

ACKNOWLEDGMENTS

So many of my patients have given me the idea for this book that all I can do is say that it is a privilege to be able to write it. I wish I had been able to give it to them sooner.

Having a good idea, however, is only a start. Stephen Hanselman saw the idea, helped me shape it until it was a gem, then got me to the right place, and stayed with it and me. He is the best. Although, I know he would say that Julia Serebrinsky is the best, and with her insight, clarity, and plain brilliance, he's probably right. Unless it's Gretchen Lees who is the best, with her ability to keep perspective, get inside my head, and help me pull out what is there in a perfect way.

I thank the entire team at Crown for their support from the start, and for dedicating themselves to making it work. Special thanks to my publisher, Tina Constable, who has led two of our projects now, with vision and care; and my editor, Sydny Miner, whose careful eye and open-mindedness are just what an author needs to do the best work and keep doing it. Heather Jackson, with her easy way, lovely touch, and great confidence, created the relationships that made this book possible and nurtured them and it perfectly.

Drs. John Petrini, Alex Soffici, Tim Rodgers, Darol Joseff, and Andy Binder and Mr. Ron Werft, all of the outstanding Santa Barbara Cottage Health System, encouraged my work every day. Ron has overseen the transformation of what might be now the best hospital food in the United States. Helmuth Billy let me bounce ideas and approaches off him even after sixteen-hour days; Samantha

Billy let us have those conversations: I am grateful, and feel like part of their family. Without the Schiedermayer family and Kim, this book would not have had David, or her generosity of spirit. Jeff Kang, now of Walgreens and formerly of Cigna, both great companies, kindly invited me to do conference menus with food as medicine in mind; Flora Ward at AARP permitted me to showcase my healthy-eating program early on in a great venue; Christopher Breuleux gave me an early chance to showcase my ideas; and Diane Goodman and Liz Piacentini of Goodman Speakers Bureau had the faith to let me try it with new audiences.

Michael DeLapa showed the kind of generosity and business insight that has made him a Silicon Valley legend (on his own terms); our friendship is older than either of us. Barbara Ficarra drew me into the snappy world of health social media, and Marc Monseau made that world bigger for me, as did Kara Blasco, Kathy Mackey, Dakila Divina of Everyday Health, and Robert Halper. Drs. Nick Genes, Jen Shine Dyer, Val Jones, and Wendy Sue Swanson all model the best of that world, of which I am privileged to be a part, and I learned more about the book's ideas from each of them. Ernesto Ramirez at Quantified Self encouraged some of the first presentations of the work. Larry Chu at Stanford Medicine X did the same, and Dennis Boyle, Alex Drane, Susannah Fox, and Donna Cryer all inspired my curiosity to discover more of how women can help men improve their health.

I have had some silent inspirations here, too: Tim Ferriss, for his clarity of purpose, entrepreneurship, and willingness to try new things; Guy Kawasaki, for his modeling of how to develop a career centered in one field, but with the curiosity to discover branches not in the textbooks; Gary Vaynerchuk, for his startup vision and love of wine; and Mari Smith, for her thoughtfulness, drive, and compassion—and of course, her Facebook insight.

I am especially indebted to my wonderful colleagues at Inky Dinky Productions, Bill and Bob Marty, and the super-talented Ellyne Lonergan, all of whom made my PBS work look and sound first-class. Bob's continued can-do spirit inspires me every time I'm on stage. I'm grateful to the former Marx Creative and staff of "Health Corner," especially David Marx and Rebecca Marx, whom I thank for introducing me to scripted TV; my colleagues there, Joan Lunden and Leeza Gibbons, I thank for showing me how it's done. Adip Thathy of Contact Designers brilliantly found the ideas and www.drjohnlapuma.com images to begin to transform this idea so it is accessible on every device. Jennifer Holland's research organization was a lifesaver. John Tomko made me think hard about exactly where this is going, and I love that focus: it made the book better.

Alan Greene, a pediatric and online pioneer, modeled for me new ways to think outside the box, and Cheryl Greene showed me how to operate inside it, even while thinking outside. Dan Nadeau, always inventive and insightful, tutored me in the intricacies of endocrinology, again.

Special thanks to the men (and the women who love them) who tested the Refuel recipes with me: you and your stories inspire me. I thank Karen Levin of Highland Park, Illinois, for her terrific recipe development and testing skills.

Karen's matchless work may just help cooking become popular for men—it is already manly. Wayne Rosing deserves special thanks: his wisdom, humility, and open-mindedness are models for all men.

Special continued thanks to Chefs Rick Bayless, Tracey Vowell, Richard James, and Geno Bahena, and the staff of Frontera Grill and Topolobampo for championing great food and commitment to local farmers. Dr. Bruce Tiffney, of the extraordinary College of Creative Studies of the University of California, Santa Barbara, kept me connected to one of the best educational institutions in the United States. Howard Gilbert was always available when I needed him, and Dr. Mehmet Oz gave me daily inspiration, in communicating in an open-hearted way exactly what needs to be said in ways his audience can hear and use. Dr. Mike Roizen, from whom I've been privileged to learn since our first book together, showed me how to develop silver linings so they shine even brighter than imaginable. Glenn Riseley of the GCC inspired sharper writing and thinking, and Elly McLean walked the talk, literally.

I thank the beautiful Annie Kratz for her kindness, love, and care, and Annie's entire family (Barbara, Steve, Tim, Anne, Kathy, Cole, Gianna, and many more), but especially Dean Kratz, whose dedication and passion have made his own Golf Mecca book world-class, and whose generosity brings together kids of all ages to chase parachutes, forty-five years running—and who let me escape to the cool recesses of air-conditioned Omaha to finish this book. Linda La Puma and Bob Anderson offered timeless encouragement and nurturance, and help make so much of my life possible.

John La Puma, MD
@johnlapuma
Santa Barbara, CA, USA
December 1, 2013

INDEX

About the Author

JOHN LA PUMA, M.D., is a board-certified specialist in internal medicine and the first physician to teach nutrition and cooking together in a U.S. medical school, with Dr. Michael Roizen. Formerly clinical associate professor of medicine at the University of Chicago Hospitals and repeatedly named "One of America's Top Physicians" by the Consumers' Research Council, Dr. La Puma has been called a "secret weapon" by the *Wall Street Journal*. He is the *New York Times* bestselling author of *ChefMD's Big Book of Culinary Medicine* and coauthor of *The RealAge Diet* and *Cooking the RealAge Way*. He is also an award-winning television host on Lifetime and PBS, founder of Refuel™, and cofounder of ChefMD®. He sees patients for weight management and nutritional concerns with Chef Clinic® in Santa Barbara, California. Subscribe to his newsletter and get free book bonuses at www.drjohnlapuma.com.

MORE FROM JOHN LA PUMA, M.D.

Doctor, What Do I Eat for That—and How Do I Make It Taste Really Good?

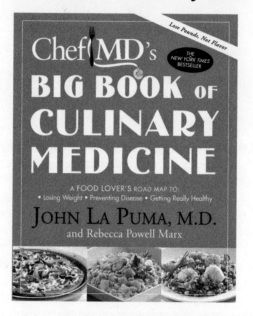

ISBN 978-0-307-39463-7

Respected physician and trained chef Dr. John La Puma answers those questions and more in this revolutionary book. In it, he offers you "culinary medicine"—the art of cooking blended with the science of medicine. The result? Restaurant-quality recipes, foods, and meals that can reverse the process of disease.

HARMONY

BOOKS • NEW YORK